The
Vita
and
Mineral
Counter

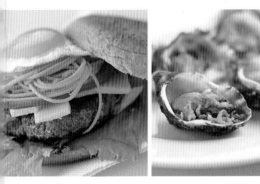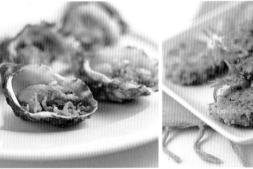

jody vassallo

Select Editions, Vancouver

VITAMINS AND MINERALS are naturally occurring substances that are essential to life. They are only needed in small amounts, but have powerful effects essential to health and well-being. They are obtained by eating a wide variety of different foods combined to make a healthy, balanced diet.

VITAMINS

These are micronutrients required for the normal functioning of all our organs, as well as functions such as growth, reproduction and tissue repair. Although they do not provide energy, they are needed for the release of energy from the macronutrients, carbohydrates, fats and proteins. With the exception of vitamins D and K, vitamins can't be made by the body and so have to be obtained through the food we eat. Vitamins can be broadly divided into two groups: fat-soluble and water-soluble.

FAT-SOLUBLE VITAMINS: These include vitamins A, D, E and K. Each have unique functions (see page 8) and occur generally in foods with a substantial fat content, such as oils, dairy products, meat, fish, nuts and grains. Because fat-soluble vitamins can be stored in the body for long periods of time, consuming large quantities can be toxic. They are fairly stable during cooking and processing, but can be destroyed by exposure to air, light or high temperatures.

WATER-SOLUBLE VITAMINS: These include vitamin C and eight B-group vitamins. These dissolve in water and so excessive amounts are generally removed from the body in the urine, although large quantities of some B vitamins (B6 and B12) can still cause toxicity problems. These vitamins can be lost in the washing, soaking or boiling of foods and may be destroyed by light or high temperatures.

MINERALS

These are essential to many processes, including maintaining the body's fluid balance and the structure of hormones, bones and teeth, the regulation of blood pressure, wound healing and the activity of muscles and nerves. Minerals cannot be made by the body, so we have to obtain them from our diet. They can be divided into two groups: major minerals and trace minerals.

MAJOR MINERALS: These include calcium, sodium, potassium, magnesium, phosphorus, chlorine and sulphur. They are classed as 'major' minerals because they are present in the body in greater amounts than the second category, trace elements.

TRACE ELEMENTS: These include iron, copper, zinc, manganese, selenium, iodine, chromium, fluoride and molybdenum. They each have different functions and cause individual deficiency symptoms if not eaten in sufficient quantities. Many other trace elements, such as boron, nickel and silicon are also found in the body, but the amounts we need to eat for optimum health are not really known.

Minerals tend to be more stable than vitamins, although the levels found in foods can be affected by food processing and preparation methods. The availability of minerals from the food we eat can be strongly affected by other nutrients (see table, top right). For example, dietary fibre can reduce the absorption of some minerals from food, whereas the lactose in milk can increase calcium absorption.

The absorption and functions of many minerals are interrelated, so a deficiency or excess of one can affect the absorption and function of others. This is why high doses of any mineral supplement should only be taken under strict medical supervision (see also 'Supplements', page 6).

MINERAL MATTERS		
Mineral	Availability/use **enhanced** by:	Availability/use **decreased** by:
Calcium	Vitamin D Regular exercise Lactose	Very high fibre intake Oxalate from spinach and rhubarb Excessive saturated fat intake
Iron	Vitamin C	Very high fibre intake Tannin (eg. in tea) Excessive zinc
Zinc	Protein Adequate energy (calories)	Very high fibre intake Excessive alcohol Excessive iron Excessive calcium
Selenium	Vitamins A, C and E	Not applicable

HOW MUCH OF EACH MINERAL AND VITAMIN DO WE NEED?

This depends on our age, gender, body size, physical activity levels, physiological status (i.e. pregnancy, breast-feeding, illness), use of medication and lifestyle factors (such as stress, smoking, exposure to pollution, alcohol and fat intake). Scientists are also trying to find out whether people with a family history of cancer, osteoporosis, heart disease and other diseases may be able to reduce their risk of developing these diseases by consuming greater amounts of certain vitamins and minerals. However, healthy people should be able to get all the vitamins and minerals they need from a balanced and varied diet.

Dietary reference values
In 1991, the UK Department of Health published Dietary Reference Values (DRVs) for Food Energy and Nutrients for the UK. DRVs is a general term for current daily dietary recommendations. Prior to the publication of this document, Recommended Daily Amounts (or RDAs) were used. RDA values were set high compared to average requirements to ensure they covered the requirements of whole groups within the population.

Although not intended for individuals, they were often wrongly used in this way. By giving a range of intakes for energy and nutrients based on the distribution of requirements, rather than just one figure, DRVs recognise the broad range of requirements of individuals within a population.

DRV is a general term that covers:
Estimated Average Requirements (EAR). This is the average requirement of a group for a particular nutrient or energy. Many people need more, and many less than the EAR.

Reference Nutrient Intake (RNI). This is the amount of a nutrient that is sufficient for almost all individuals. This level of intake is higher than most people need.

Lower Reference Nutrient Intake (LRNI). This is the amount of a nutrient that is sufficient for only a few individuals with low needs. Most people need more than the LRNI.

Safe Intake. This is a range of intakes sufficient for almost all individuals' needs, but not high enough to cause undesirable effects. This is given for nutrients where there is currently insufficient information to estimate requirements precisely.

DRVs give a general guide to whether or not an individual's diet is likely to be nutritionally adequate. This book gives RNIs for most vitamins and minerals, as this is the level likely to be adequate for most people.

OPTIMUM INTAKES
Nutrient intake in relation to health is sometimes described in the following way: deficient, adequate, optimal, excessive, toxic. RNIs are usually set at a level to prevent deficiency. An 'optimal' intake refers to a level of intake that not only prevents deficiency, but also that may positively improve health or protect us from disease. Scientists are currently unable to calculate RNIs for optimal health and do not recommend the regular consumption of high dose vitamin and mineral supplements.

FOOD LABELS
The RNIs used in the UK are calculated from studies of physiological requirements of healthy people. But, because these studies are subject to interpretation, the RNI values for a nutrient can vary from country to country (eg. RNIs are lower in the UK than in the USA). European Union regulations require that RDAs be shown on food and supplement labels that are sold in the UK. RDAs only apply to 'average adults' and only give a rough guide to requirement. They are not the same as RNIs.

GETTING THE VITAMINS AND MINERALS YOU NEED FROM A HEALTHY DIET
The diagram on the right shows the types of foods and the proportions we should eat them in to have a healthy, balanced diet containing the vitamins and minerals we need.

Breads, other cereals and potatoes
At least half of the calories we eat should come from the starchy foods included in this group. Because they're bulky, low in fat and often high in fibre, these foods fill us up without providing too many calories. It tends to be what you serve with them (eg. butter on bread or high-fat sauces on pasta) that adds the fat and calories. This group also includes breakfast cereals, oats, pasta, noodles, plantains, beans and lentils. These foods provide carbohydrate (starch), some calcium and iron and B vitamins.

Fruit and vegetables
Eat plenty of these foods – at least five portions a day. Choose from a variety of fresh, frozen or canned fruits and vegetables. These foods are packed with antioxidant vitamins, especially vitamin C and carotenes (vitamin A), as well as folates, fibre and some carbohydrates. They are also low in fat and calories.

Milk and dairy products
Eat moderate amounts of these foods and choose lower fat alternatives where possible. This group includes milk, cheese, yoghurt and fromage frais, but it does not include butter, eggs and cream. Milk and dairy products provide calcium, protein, vitamins B12, A and D. Although semi-skimmed and skimmed milk contain less of the fat-soluble vitamins A and D, their calcium content is the same as full-fat milk.

Meat, fish and alternatives
Eat moderate amounts of these foods and choose low-fat alternatives where possible. This group also includes eggs, nuts, textured vegetable protein, tofu, beans and lentils. Eat at least two portions of fish every week, one of which should be an oily fish. Oily fish contain omega-3 fatty acids, which may help reduce the tendency for blood to clot, reducing the risk of heart disease. These foods provide iron, protein, B vitamins, zinc and magnesium.

Foods containing fat and/or sugar
Eat these types of foods sparingly and choose lower fat alternatives where possible. This group includes butter, other fat spreads, oils, salad dressings and treats, such as biscuits, cakes, chocolate, ice cream, sweets, crisps and sweetened drinks. Sugary foods should be limited as frequent consumption can lead to tooth decay.

HOW TO EAT A HEALTHY DIET

To ensure you get all the nutrients you need for a healthy diet, you should eat a wide variety of different foods and:

• Eat a low-fat diet, where no more than 35 per cent of the calories you eat comes from fat. For men (at a healthy weight) eating 2500 calories a day, this is equivalent to 95 g fat per day. For women (at a healthy weight) eating 2000 calories a day, this is equivalent to 75 g fat per day.

• Replace saturated fat in your diet with unsaturates, particularly monounsaturates. No more than about 10 per cent of the calories you eat should be from saturated fat. Fat in food contains a mixture of saturated, monounsaturated and polyunsaturated fat, but one type usually predominates. One way to eat less saturates is to eat less total fat.

• Increase intake of n-3 polyunsaturates (omega-3 fatty acids) by eating at least 2 portions of fish every week, one of which should be an oily variety.

• Make sure that half of the calories you eat comes from starchy carbohydrates, such as potatoes, bread, rice, pasta and other cereals. For most of us, this means eating at least half as much again of these foods.

• Eat at least five portions of fruit and vegetables every day.

• Eat plenty of fibre (about 18 g) every day. This includes the soluble fibre found in oats, pulses, fruit and vegetables, as well as the insoluble fibre found in wholemeal bread, wholemeal pasta, wholegrain rice and wholewheat breakfast cereals.

• Drink sensibly. Women should drink no more than 2–3 units of alcohol every day and men 3–4 units per day. These are maximum limits, but it's best to keep under these daily benchmarks.

• Eat less salt (sodium chloride). Most of the salt we eat comes from processed,

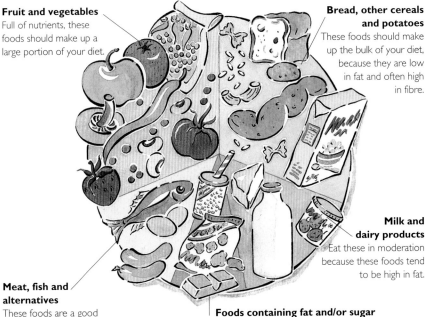

Fruit and vegetables
Full of nutrients, these foods should make up a large portion of your diet.

Bread, other cereals and potatoes
These foods should make up the bulk of your diet, because they are low in fat and often high in fibre.

Milk and dairy products
Eat these in moderation because these foods tend to be high in fat.

Meat, fish and alternatives
These foods are a good source of protein, but are best eaten in moderation.

Foods containing fat and/or sugar
Limit your intake of these foods because they can lead to obesity and tooth decay.

manufactured foods rather than the salt we add during cooking or at the table.
• Don't have sugary foods and drinks too often. They contain calories but few nutrients and may contribute to overweight and tooth decay.

GETTING THE MOST FROM YOUR FOOD

Although we tend to think that modern foods are depleted in vitamins and minerals, supermarkets are actually full of nutritious foods – fresh, frozen and dried. Vitamins and minerals are even added to some processed foods to replace those that are lost during the manufacturing process (eg. fortified breakfast cereals and bread), or to increase the nutrient content of food (eg. some milks and fat spreads). There are ways to retain more of the nutrients in the meals you prepare:
• When you buy fresh fruit and vegetables, ensure they are as fresh as possible and eat them within a few days. Store in a cool, dark, dry place for the shortest possible time.
• To retain more vitamins, blanch and freeze fruit and vegetables from fresh.
• When preparing fruit and vegetables, cut them with a sharp knife and do not slice too finely. Where possible, try to leave the skin on. In potatoes, for example, most of the vitamin C is found just beneath the skin.
• Eat vegetables raw, or if you are going to cook them, prepare them just before cooking. Microwaving or stir-frying retains more nutrients than boiling. Cook all vegetables for the shortest time and in a small amount of water. If boiling, bring the water to the boil first, cut up the vegetables, then add them to the water. Vitamin C and B are easily destroyed during boiling. They leach out into the cooking water.
• Eat food straight away once cooked. Keeping food warm for 15 minutes, for example, could reduce the vitamin C content by 25 per cent.
• Fresh fruit and vegetables aren't always better than canned or frozen. Canned beans, for example, contain similar levels of nutrients to home-cooked dried beans; quickly reheated frozen peas contain more

nutrients than overcooked (or old) fresh ones.
• Do not use bicarbonate of soda when cooking (sometimes done to help retain green colour of vegetables). It destroys vitamin C.

SUPPLEMENTS

At the moment, it's safe to say that the perfect supplement does not exist, but it is clear that a balanced diet offers many health benefits. Whole foods are a complex package of nutrients and other beneficial factors that are not found in supplements. For example, an orange contains vitamin C with carotene, folate, calcium, fibre and possibly other bio-active compounds that may protect our health. You won't get all of these elements in a vitamin C supplement. Apart from tasting better, here are some other reasons why we should get our nutrients from food rather than supplements:
• Other components in food (not present in supplements) can increase nutrient absorption in the body.
• The chemical form of a nutrient may be different from the natural form and may not be absorbed as well.
• High-dose supplements can reduce absorption of other nutrients.
• Taking excessive amounts of some nutrients may have toxic effects, or in the case of some water-soluble vitamins, the excess may just be excreted in the urine.
• Foods also contain other bio-active compounds (or phytochemicals) that have antioxidant properties and may help protect us against cancer, heart disease and diabetes.

When are supplements needed?

In some circumstances, vitamin and mineral supplements may be needed to improve your health or to prevent a health problem from developing. There are two reasons why you may not get all the nutrients you need from your diet: either you don't eat enough or you don't absorb enough. Some people don't get all the nutrients they need from their diet, because they don't eat a healthy balance of foods or because they have a greater nutrient requirement (eg. during pregnancy, illness or high activity levels). Also, high intakes of fat, alcohol and certain medications can increase the body's use of certain vitamins and minerals, while some illnesses and medications prevent them from being absorbed.

While most people can get all the vitamins and minerals they need from a healthy diet, some groups of people may benefit from certain supplements:
• Folic acid is recommended for women planning to have a baby. They should take 400 mcg folic acid every day until the end of the twelfth week of pregnancy to reduce the risk of the baby being born with neural tube defects.
• Vitamin D may be needed for children under the age of four, pregnant and breast-feeding women, and people over 65 years if they don't include much meat and fish in their diet. It may also be required by people who rarely go outdoors (eg. are housebound or in residential care) or those who wear very concealing clothing. Some young African-Caribbean children who have a very strict vegan diet, and babies, children and women from some Asian communities may need extra vitamin D.
• Vitamin drops containing vitamins A, C and D are recommended for children under the age of five as a safeguard for when their diets may be insufficient. You should start giving your baby vitamin drops (available at low cost from health centres) at six months old, if you are still breast-feeding or when your baby has less than one pint of infant formula every day. Ask your health visitor for advice.

Also, if you fit into any of the following categories, you may benefit from taking some supplements and should seek medical advice:
• Women with regular heavy periods may need iron supplements.
• If you are a heavy smoker or drinker, you may benefit from supplements eg. vitamin C and some B vitamins.
• If you are removing whole food groups from your diet due to allergy or intolerance.

For example, avoiding all dairy products may mean you need extra calcium and vitamin D.
• If you have a strict vegan diet, you may need extra iron, vitamin B12 and vitamin D.
• If you have a low-calorie weight-loss diet, you may need extra iron, calcium and zinc.
• If you are taking certain long-term medications, they may interfere with the absorption of some nutrients.

If you are healthy and you want to take a supplement, choose a multi-vitamin/mineral variety, providing RNI amounts or less.

USING THE TABLES
This book contains charts and tables, one for each vitamin and most minerals, listing foods that are good sources of these nutrients. Each chart states the adult RNI (where applicable) and lists the average amount of vitamin or mineral contained in 100 g of the edible part of the food. Vitamins and minerals are only present in foods (and needed in the body) in small amounts, for example, milligrams (mg) or micrograms (mcg).

The tables will help you estimate the nutrient content of your diet and thus improve your eating habits by making better food choices and meeting the RNI. All nutrient values are for the raw, uncooked food unless otherwise stated. In most cases, the nutrient content shown is the average amount found in the UK variety of the food. However, if UK food data was not available, Australian sources were used. Foods at the top of the lists contain relatively high amounts of the nutrient per 100 g. Although not all of these foods are eaten in large amounts, such as yeast extract or wheat bran, they can make a valuable contribution to your nutrient intake if eaten regularly. On the other hand, some of the foods at the bottom of the lists (which contain lower levels of the particular nutrient) may be eaten in larger amounts, such as potatoes and pasta, and therefore also make a significant contribution to your nutrient intake. Potatoes, for example, account for about 35 per cent of the vitamin C intake in the UK. Some of the recipe ideas and suggestions accompanying the lists will give you examples of how to incorporate these foods into your daily diet.

VITAMINS

FAT-SOLUBLE

	RNI	FUNCTION
VITAMIN A	Females 11+ years: 600 mcg RE*/day. Pregnancy: 700 mcg RE/day. Lactation: 950 mcg RE/day. Males 15+ years: 700 mcg RE/day. Do not exceed: 7500 mcg RE/day (females); pregnant women, see page 22; 9000 mcg RE/day (males).	For reproduction and development. Required for healthy skin, eyes and hair. Helps the body resist infection and maintains healthy mucous membranes.
VITAMIN D	No RNI except females and males 65+ years: 10 mcg/day. Pregnancy and lactation: 10 mcg/day. Vitamin D is made when skin is exposed to sunlight.	Needed for calcium and phosphorus absorption and for healthy bones and teeth.
VITAMIN E	Safe intake:+ Men above 4 mg/day. Women above 3mg/day.	Natural antioxidant, helps healing, prevents scarring. Keeps nerves and red blood cells healthy. Protects cell membranes.
VITAMIN K	Safe intake: Adults 1 mcg/kg body weight/day. Most of the body's vitamin K is synthesised by intestinal bacteria, only about 20 per cent is obtained from foods.	Called the band-aid vitamin, promotes blood clotting to stop bleeding.
OTHER FAT-SOLUBLE NUTRIENTS	.Approximately 1 per cent of total energy (kj/cal) intake.	Needed for normal development and growth, and healthy skin and eyes.
ESSENTIAL FATTY ACIDS	No RNI	

* **RE** Dietary vitamin A (or retinol) is measured in retinol equivalents (RE) because, as well as the ready-formed vitamin A in foods of animal origin, beta carotene (sometimes called pro-vitamin A) in plant foods is converted to retinol in the body. 6 mcg of beta carotene is equivalent to 1 mcg retinol. So RE represents the retinol present in the foods plus the vitamin A that will be made in the body from the beta carotene.

DEFICIENCY SIGNS	FOOD SOURCES	SYNERGISTS	ABSORPTION INHIBITORS
Poor vision, dry scaly skin, impaired reproduction and growth, increased susceptibility to infection.	Liver, fish, eggs, dairy products (eg. milk and cheese). Yellow, orange, red and dark green vegetables contain large amounts of beta carotene eg. dried apricots, sweet potato, mangoes, carrots, spinach, watercress.	Zinc, vitamin D.	Colestipol, Cholestyramine, Epsom salts, some antibiotics, alcohol, a very low fat intake.
Muscle and bone weakness. Rickets in children. Osteomalacia in adults.	Kippers, mackerel, salmon, canned sardines, herrings, tuna, prawns, milk, butter, fortified margarines, egg yolk, fish oils.	Vitamin A, calcium and phosphorus.	Alcohol, some antibiotics, olestra, mineral oil, laxatives, some anticonvulsants.
Rare. Can occur in premature babies and people on very low-fat diets. Red blood cells may rupture, poor wound healing.	Wheat germ oil, sunflower seeds, sunflower oil, safflower oil, peanut oil, olive oil, almonds, peanuts, hazelnuts, eggs, green leafy vegetables and wholegrains.	Vitamin C.	Metals, heat, oxygen, freezing, processing, large intakes of vitamin K, Epsom salts, laxatives, senokot.
Abnormal blood clotting, haemorrhaging. Deficiency is rare in adults but can occur in newborn babies.	Green leafy vegetables (eg. broccoli, kale, Brussels sprouts, cabbage and Swiss chard), milk, liver, wheat bran, oats, vegetable oils.	Vitamin C.	Unstable to heat, freezing, warfarin, x-rays, radiation, air pollution, some antibiotics, mineral oil, laxatives, large doses of vitamin E.
Impaired vision and hearing, growth failure in infants, dry scaly skin, poor wound healing.	Oily fish, cold-pressed vegetable oils, nuts, hazelnuts, prawns, salmon, soya beans.	Vitamin E.	Not applicable.

✝ **alpha-tocopherol** is the most prevalent form of vitamin E, but you may see it listed as 'mixed tocopherols' on food labels and supplements.

VITAMINS
WATER-SOLUBLE

	RNI	FUNCTION
VITAMIN B1 THIAMIN	Females 15+ years: 0.8 mg/day. Pregnancy: 0.9 mg/day. Lactation: 1.0 mg/day. Males 19–50 years 1.0 mg/day. Males 51+ years 0.9 mg/day. Consuming over 3 g/day over a long period may have undesirable effects.	Needed for converting food into energy, growth in childhood and fertility in adults. Maintains healthy heart and nervous system.
VITAMIN B2 RIBOFLAVIN	Females 11+ years: 1.1 mg/day. Pregnancy: 1.4 mg/day. Lactation: 1.6 mg/day. Males 15+ years: 1.3 mg/day.	Helps the body release energy from food. Promotes growth, also needed for healthy eyes, hair, skin and nails.
VITAMIN B3 NIACIN★	Females 19–50 years: 13 mg NE/day. Females 51+ years: 12 mg NE/day. No extra needed during pregnancy. Lactation: 15 mg NE/day. Males 19–50 years: 17 mg NE/day. Males 51+ years: 16 mg/day.	Needed to release energy from food. Involved in controlling blood sugar, keeping skin healthy and maintaining healthy nervous and digestive systems.
VITAMIN B5 PANTOTHENIC ACID	No RNI. Current UK intakes of 3–7 mg/day are considered adequate.	Helps the body release energy from food. Aids the formation of antibodies and maintains a healthy nervous system and skin.
VITAMIN B6 PYRIDOXINE	Females 15+ years: 1.2 mg/day. No extra needed during pregnancy or lactation. Males 19+ years: 1.4 mg/day. Very high intakes (between 50 mg/day and 7 g/day) have been associated with impaired function of the sensory nerves.	Essential for protein metabolism, forming red blood cells, antibodies and neurotransmitters (brain chemicals).

★ The related compounds – nicotinic acid and nicotinamide – are both called niacin. In addition to the preformed vitamin occurring in food, one of the essential amino acids tryptophan can be converted in the body to niacin. Total vitamin activity (expressed as niacin equivalent – NE) is derived from preformed vitamin plus the amount made in the body from tryptophan.

DEFICIENCY SIGNS	FOOD SOURCES	SYNERGISTS	ABSORPTION INHIBITORS
Muscle fatigue, poor concentration, irritability, depression, heart problems. Severe deficiency: beri-beri.	Yeast extract, brown rice, porridge, wheat germ, pulses, nuts, seeds, lean meats (especially pork), offal, wholegrain products, fortified breakfast cereals.	Other B vitamins, sulphur.	Can be destroyed by cooking, storage or processing. Sensitive to oxygen, heat, low-acid conditions. Alcohol, sulphur drugs, some antibiotics, antacids, tea, coffee, blueberries, red cabbage, water.
Poor wound healing, sore, watery bloodshot eyes, cracked lips and corners of the mouth, flaking skin, rash between nose and lips, confusion.	Yeast extract, milk, cheese, yoghurt, eggs, meat, offal (eg. liver), green leafy vegetables, fortified breakfast cereals.	Other B vitamins.	Destroyed by heat and light. Oral contraceptive pill, alcohol, sulphur drugs, some tranquillisers and antidepressants.
Rare. Dermatitis, nausea, diarrhoea, muscular weakness, depression, dementia. Severe deficiency: pellagra – bright red tongue, headaches.	Yeast extract, pork, chicken, beef, fish, nuts, cheese, milk, eggs, bread, potatoes, pasta, rice and fortified breakfast cereals.	Other B vitamins, especially B6, vitamin C.	B2 is the most stable B vitamin. Sulphur drugs, alcohol, food processing.
Rare and hard to diagnose. May occur in conjunction with other B deficiencies.	Dried yeast, liver, yeast extract, kidney, nuts, wheat germ, soya flour, brown rice, eggs, pulses, wholemeal bread,	Other B vitamins.	Exposure to heat. Food processing, canning, caffeine, sulphur drugs, antibiotics, alcohol.
Depression, headaches, confusion, numbness and tingling in hands and feet, anaemia, skin lesions, poor growth, decreased antibody formation (immunity).	Dried yeast, yeast extract, wholemeal bread, wheat germ, wheatbran, fortified breakfast cereals, liver, avocados, bananas, fish, meat, nuts.	Vitamins B1, B2, B5.	Exposure to heat and light. Prolonged storage, food processing, roasting and stewing meats, alcohol, oral contraceptive pill, smoking, some antibiotics, light, air, alkaline conditions.

VITAMINS
WATER-SOLUBLE

	RNI	FUNCTION
VITAMIN B12 COBALAMIN	Females and males 15+ years 1.5 mcg/day. No extra required during pregnancy. Lactation 2.0 mcg/day.	Forms and regenerates red blood cells, needed for DNA synthesis, maintains a healthy nervous system, needed for energy production.
FOLATE OR FOLIC ACID	Females and males 11+ years 200 mcg/day. Pregnancy 300 mcg/day (see also page 44). Lactation 260 mcg/day.	Works with B12 to protect and develop the nervous system and production of genetic material. Production of red blood cells for babies in utero. Protects against birth defects.
VITAMIN C ASCORBIC ACID	Females and males 15+ years 40 mg/day. Pregnancy 50 mg/day. Lactation 70 mg/day.	Collagen production, required for healthy, skin, bones, cartilage, teeth and blood vessels. Promotes healing, aids iron absorption. Also as a powerful antioxidant.
BIOTIN	No RNI. Intakes between 10 and 200 mcg/day are considered adequate and safe.	Essential for energy production and fat and protein metabolism. Needed for healthy skin and hair, and production of sex hormones.

OTHER WATER-SOLUBLE NUTRIENTS

FLAVONOIDS	No RNI.	Powerful antioxidants thought to reduce risk of chronic diseases like heart disease and cancer.
INOSITOL	No RNI. Can be made in the body from glucose.	Involved in relaying messages to the inside of cells. Combines with choline (see below) to form lecithin.
CHOLINE	No RNI. Can easily be made in the body.	Involved in cholesterol and fat metabolism, production of neuro-transmitters, promotes healthy cell membranes.

DEFICIENCY SIGNS	FOOD SOURCES	SYNERGISTS	ABSORPTION INHIBITORS
Pernicious anaemia, nerve problems.	Liver, heart, kidney, meat, poultry, fish, milk, cheese, eggs, fortified breakfast cereals.	Folate.	Exposure to air, light and vitamin C, antacids, laxatives, oral contraceptive pill, alcohol, anticonvulsants.
Anaemia, apathy, depression, swollen painful tongue, poor growth, problems with nerve development and functioning.	Dried yeast, liver, dark green leafy vegetables (eg. broccoli and cabbage), pulses, nuts, oat bran, yeast extract.	Other B vitamins especially B12 and B6, and vitamin C.	Exposure to air, light, heat and acidic conditions, alcohol, contraceptive pill, analgesics (aspirin), some antibiotics, anticonvulsants.
Loss of appetite, muscle cramps, dry skin, splitting hair, bleeding gums, bruising, nosebleeds, anaemia, infections, slow healing.	Citrus fruits, blackcurrants, strawberries, kiwi fruit, papaya, red chillies, broccoli, watercress, parsley, green leafy vegetables, red and green peppers.	Vitamin E, selenium.	Heat, light, oxygen, exposure to copper and iron cookware, bicarbonate of soda, contraceptive pill, anticonvulsants, analgesics.
Uncommon. Lethargy, nausea, thinning of hair, loss of hair colour, red skin rash, depression.	Brewer's yeast, liver, yeast extract, pulses, nuts, whole wheat, brown rice, milk, cheese, yoghurt, eggs.	Other B vitamins, sulphur.	Raw egg white, food processing, sulphur drugs. (Sulphur and biotin are synergists but they compete for absorption.)
Not known.	Most fruits and vegetables including citrus fruit (especially pith), buckwheat.	Vitamin C.	Water, cooking, heat, light, oxygen.
Raised cholesterol levels, nerve disorders, intestinal problems.	Wheat germ, cereals and pulses, oranges, peanuts.	Other B vitamins, choline.	Food processing, alcohol, coffee.
Rare. Unlikely in healthy people. Causes liver problems.	Eggs, egg yolks, liver, kidney, brain, lettuce, leafy green vegetables, wheat bran and germ, pulses.	Other B vitamins, inositol.	Food processing, alcohol.

MINERALS
MAJOR MINERALS

MAJOR MINERALS	RNI	FUNCTION
CALCIUM	Females and males 19+ years: 700 mg/day. No extra needed for pregnancy due to increased absorption. Lactation: 1250 mg/day.	Maintains strong bones and teeth, regulates nerve and muscle function, required for blood clotting and blood pressure regulation, enzyme regulation.
MAGNESIUM	Females 19+ years: 270 mg/day. No extra needed for pregnancy due to increased absorption. Lactation: 320 mg/day. Males 15+ years: 300 mg/day.	In combination with phosphorus and sodium, required for muscle and nerve function. Needed for energy. Maintains bone structure, regulates calcium balance.
PHOSPHORUS	Females and males 19+ years: 550 mg/day. No extra needed for pregnancy due to increased absorption. Lactation: 990 mg/day Do not exceed 70 mg/kg body weight/day.	With calcium and magnesium, maintains bone structure. Needed for the production of energy in all body cells.
SODIUM	Females and males 15+ years: 1600 mg/day (equivalent to about 4g salt or sodium chloride). No extra needed for pregnancy or lactation. More than 3.2 g/day (about 8 g salt) may lead to raised blood pressure.	Works with potassium to regulate fluid and acid/alkali balance in the body and therefore responsible for nerve and muscle function.
POTASSIUM	Females and males 15+ years: 3500 mg/day. No extra needed for pregnancy or lactation.	Works with sodium to regulate the body's fluid balance, maintains normal blood pressure and heartbeat and nerve impulses.
CHLORIDE	Females and males 15+ years: 2500 mg/day. No extra needed for pregnancy or lactation.	Works with sodium and potassium to regulate acid/alkali and water balance.

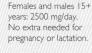

DEFICIENCY SIGNS	FOOD SOURCES	SYNERGISTS	ABSORPTION INHIBITORS
Osteoporosis, osteomalacia, muscle spasms and cramping, rickets, high blood pressure, heart palpitations, joint pain.	Dairy products, canned fish eg. sardines and salmon eaten with their bones, some breakfast cereals, sesame seeds, almonds, green leafy vegetables, fortified soya milk and tofu.	Vitamin D, inositol, phosphorus, magnesium.	High phosphorus, salt or protein intake. Alcohol, oxalic acid (in chocolate, rhubarb), phytate eg. in bran, some laxatives, some diuretics, some antibiotics, large doses B complex pills.
Rare. Nausea, anxiety, muscle spasms, cramps, tremors, changes in blood pressure and heartbeat.	Nuts, soya beans, brewer's yeast, wholemeal bread and pasta, peas, seafood, dried fruit, seeds.	Calcium, vitamin D, phosphorus.	Alcohol, calcium carbonate antacid, some antibiotics, some diuretics.
Rare. Muscle weakness, bone pain, rickets, osteoporosis.	Meat, fish, dairy products, nuts, wheat bran, pumpkin, sunflower seeds, sesame seeds.	Calcium, magnesium, vitamin D.	Excess magnesium and aluminium.
Rare, can occur with chronic diarrhoea, vomiting, excess sweating.	Table salt, cured meats (eg. bacon), smoked fish, sauces, olives, canned food in brine, highly processed foods, cheese, butter, fatty snack foods, mineral waters.	Potassium, chloride.	Some diuretics, anti-gout drugs, some antibiotics, some laxatives.
Rare, can occur with chronic diarrhoea, vomiting, excess sweating. Confusion, cramps, fatigue, irregular heartbeat, extreme thirst.	Fresh fruit and vegetables (eg. apples, bananas, carrots, potatoes, broccoli, dates, oranges), wheat bran, fish, meat, poultry, milk and yoghurt.	Sodium, chloride.	Excess sodium, alcohol, coffee, some diuretics, some laxatives, some antibiotics, anti-gout drugs.
Rare.	Table salt, olives, tomato sauce, bacon, canned fish, cheese, peanuts, processed foods containing salt.	Sodium, potassium.	Not applicable.

MINERALS
MAJOR MINERALS

		RNI	FUNCTION
SULPHUR	S	No RNI. Most comes from the proteins we eat.	Essential for healthy hair, skin and nails. Needed for protein synthesis and for detoxifying drugs and protecting cells from oxidative damage.

MINERALS
TRACE MINERALS

		RNI	FUNCTION
IRON	Fe	Females 11–50 years: 14.8 mg/day. Females 50+ years: 8.7mg/day. Males 19+ years: 8.7 mg/day. No extra usually needed for pregnancy or lactation.	Oxygen transport and storage in muscles, improves immunity, required for growth, energy production, drug metabolism and proper mental functioning.
ZINC		Females 15+ years: 7 mg/day. No extra required during pregnancy. Lactation: 0–4 months 13 mg/day. 4+ months 9.5 mg/day. Male 15+ years: 9.5 mg/day. Acute intake of 2 g zinc produces nausea. Regularly consuming more than 50 mg/day may interfere with copper metabolism.	Improves immunity, healing. Needed for healthy eyes, skin, nails, for growth and sexual development, for the activity of enzymes, for DNA and protein synthesis, and activity of vitamins A and D.
COPPER	Cu	Females and males 19+ years: 1.2 mg/day. No extra needed during pregnancy. Lactation: 1.5 mg/day. High intakes are harmful. In some countries, levels of 1.6 mg per litre in drinking water have been associated with toxic effects.	Needed for iron and fat metabolism, connective tissue synthesis, maintenance of the heart muscle, functioning of the nervous and immune systems, maintains red blood cell membranes.

DEFICIENCY SIGNS	FOOD SOURCES	SYNERGISTS	ABSORPTION INHIBITORS
Rare. Usually only occurs with a diet that is very low in protein.	Eggs, meat, chicken, fish, seafood, kidney, heart, liver, spinach, nuts, Brussels sprouts, bread, cheese, dried fruits.	Thiamin, biotin.	Not applicable.
Anaemia, reduced physical and mental performance, fatigue, poor circulation, depression, decreased resistance to infection and illness.	Red meat, liver, clams, mussels, oysters, chicken, fish, eggs, spinach and other green leafy vegetables, dried apricots, cocoa powder, fortified breakfast cereals, wholemeal bread.	Vitamin C.	Phytate (seeds, nuts, grains), large quantities tea/coffee, calcium supplements, analgesics (aspirin), narcotics (codeine, morphine), some antacids, some antibiotics and anti-gout drugs.
White spots on nails, loss of taste and appetite, poor growth and wound healing, night blindness, late onset of puberty, dry flaky skin, dandruff, increased susceptibility to infection.	Oysters, crab and shellfish, other seafood, red meat, chicken, liver, dairy products, some green vegetables, eggs, nuts and wheat germ.	Vitamin A, vitamin D, copper.	Alcohol, some diuretics, some drugs, oral contraceptive pill, hormone replacement therapy, phytate (seeds, nuts, grains), large amounts of tea, coffee, diet high in iron, iron supplements.
Uncommon. Anaemia, decreased immunity, blood vessel and bone weakening, red blood cell damage, arthritis, impaired growth, and heart muscle and nervous system degeneration.	Shellfish (oysters, lobster, crab), offal (eg. liver), nuts and seeds, wholegrains, prunes, soya products.	Zinc, iron.	High zinc diet. Zinc supplements. High intake of iron. (Copper, zinc and iron are synergists, but compete for absorption.) High intake of manganese, molybdenum, vitamin C and antacids.

MINERALS
TRACE MINERALS

	RNI	FUNCTION
MANGANESE Mn	Safe intake: Adults more than 1.4 mg/day.	Functions together with zinc and copper in a major antioxidant compound. Involved in carbohydrate and fat metabolism and brain function.
IODINE I	Females and males 15+ years: 140 mcg/day. No extra needed for pregnancy or lactation. Do not exceed 17 mcg/kg/day (or 1000 mcg/day). Excessively high intake may cause hyperthyroidism.	Essential component of the thyroid hormones which regulate metabolic rate, growth and development, and promote protein synthesis.
CHROMIUM Cr	Safe intake:. Adults more than 25 mcg/day.	Needed for insulin to function normally and for glucose to enter cells. Involved in fat and protein metabolism.
MOLYBDENUM	Safe intake: Adults 50–400 mcg/day.	Required for enzymes involved in producing waste products before they are excreted (detoxification), and oxidation and detoxification of many other compounds.
FLUORIDE F	No RNI or safe intake for adults.	Prevents tooth decay and discolouration, strengthens bones.
SELENIUM	Females 15+ years: 60 mcg/day. No extra needed for pregnancy. Lactation: 75 mcg/day. Males 19+ years: 75 mcg/day.	Works with vitamin E in an antioxidant enzyme. Needed for synthesis of thyroid hormones which regulate basal metabolic rate.

DEFICIENCY SIGNS	FOOD SOURCES	SYNERGISTS	ABSORPTION INHIBITORS
Rare. Growth retardation, bone abnormalities, brain and reproductive function problems, fat and carbohydrate metabolism problems.	Nuts, sesame seeds, wheat germ, wheat bran, oat bran, legumes, blackberries, spinach.	Copper, zinc.	Not applicable.
Goitre (enlarged thyroid gland, swelling in the neck), metabolic rate drops, bulging eyes, fatigue, mental retardation, hair loss, slow reflexes, dry skin.	Iodised salt, seafood (eg. clams, haddock, oysters, salmon, sardines), dairy products, eggs, seaweed.	Selenium.	Goitrogen substances in foods (turnips, cabbage, cassava, Brussels sprouts).
High blood glucose and insulin levels. High blood cholesterol and triglyceride levels.	Egg yolk, red meat, liver, dairy products, whole grains, nuts, potato, oysters, clams, rye bread, wine, chillies, spinach, oranges, apple peel, wholegrain bread.		Not applicable.
Rare, only seen in hospital patients on deficient feed tubes. Impaired growth, reduced appetite.	Grains, legumes, dairy products, spinach, cauliflower, peas, corn, kidneys, liver.		Not applicable.
Increased tooth decay, particularly up to the age of 13 years.	Fluoridated water, tea, fish eaten with bones, milk, Cheddar cheese. Also fluoridated toothpaste.	Calcium.	Aluminium cookware.
Seen in areas with low selenium soil levels. Muscular aches and weakness. A form of heart disease called Keshan disease.	Seafood, liver, kidney, eggs, meat, wholegrains, brazil nuts, wheat germ, wholegrain bread.	Vitamin E, iodine	Not applicable.

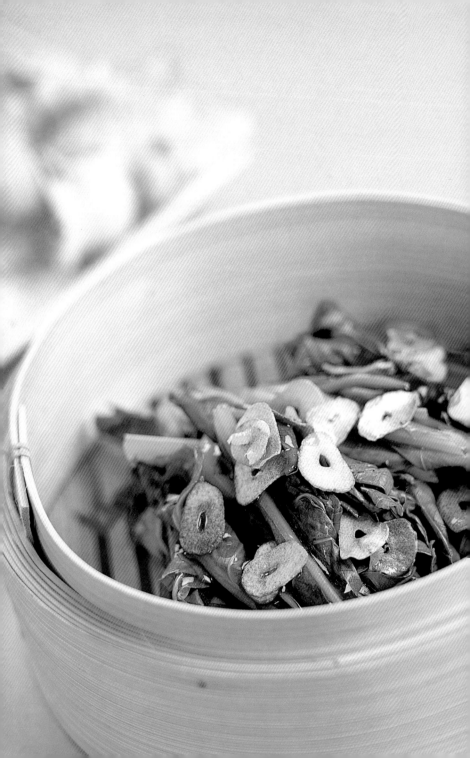

vitamins
and other
nutrients

FAT-SOLUBLE VITAMINS

FAT-SOLUBLE NUTRIENTS

WATER-SOLUBLE VITAMINS

OTHER WATER-SOLUBLE NUTRIENTS

VITAMINS – FAT-SOLUBLE
VITAMIN A

REFERENCE NUTRIENT INTAKE
Men: 700 mcg RE[+]/day Women: 600 mcg RE/day
(+ RE see page 8)

FOOD SOURCES	mcg RE per 100 g
Liver, calf, fried	25200
Liver, lamb, fried	19700
Liver, chicken, fried	10500
Pâté, liver	7400
Carrots, raw	1353
Carrots, boiled	1260
Low fat spread	1084
Margarine	905
Butter	887
Sweet potato, baked	855
Red chillies	685
Parsley	673
Double cream	654
Red peppers (capsicum)	640
Spinach, boiled	640
Butternut squash, baked	548
Cream cheese	422
Watercress	420
Mixed frozen vegetables, boiled	420
Spring greens, boiled	378
Hard cheese	373
Tomatoes, grilled	307
Mangoes	300
Chicken eggs, whole, cooked or raw	190
Papaya (pawpaw)	165
Canteloupe melon	165
Greek yoghurt	121
Tomatoes	107
Apricots, dried	105
Broccoli, boiled	80
Milk, whole	56

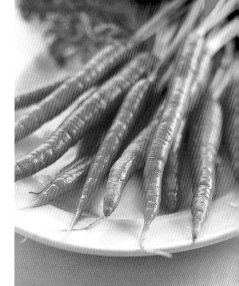

Vitamin A is essential for good vision, hence the belief that carrots are good for your eyesight. Vitamin A requirement may be increased if you strain your eyes watching too much television, working in poor light or glare, or looking at a computer screen all day.

RECIPE Combine slices of a fresh ripe mango, chunks of canteloupe melon, some finely shredded ginger, chopped dried apricots, hazelnuts and sprigs of fresh mint. Drizzle with a little lime juice and sprinkle with cinnamon. This is a great way to start the day with vitamin A.

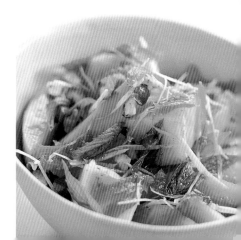

RECIPE Marinate chicken livers in a Japanese-style teriyaki marinade, then thread them onto skewers and barbecue or grill them.

A glass of carrot and ginger juice is an excellent source of carotenoids for those who eat breakfast on the run.

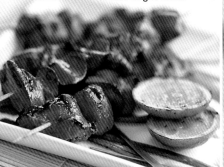
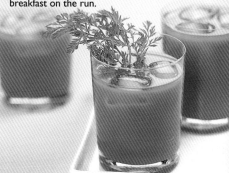

VITAMIN A is a fat-soluble vitamin and comes in two forms:

PREFORMED VITAMIN A (retinoids) that we obtain from foods of animal origin, such as liver and dairy products.

PROVITAMIN A (beta-carotene and other carotenoids) which can be converted to active vitamin A in the body, and comes from red and yellow fruits, dark green leafy vegetables, and vegetables such as carrots (from which they derive their name).

Vitamin A is essential for good vision, assists the growth and repair of body tissues and helps maintain soft skin and hair. Beta carotene is a powerful antioxidant vitamin.

Approximately one third of the carotene in food is converted to vitamin A. Light cooking, puréeing and mashing ruptures the cell membrane and makes the carotene more readily available.

CAUTION Vitamin A can build up to toxic levels. Don't exceed 9000 mcg RE/day (men); 7500 mcg RE/day (women). Vitamin A supplements (including any fish oil supplements high in vitamin A) should be avoided by pregnant women and people who are taking vitamin A acne preparations or broad-spectrum antibiotics. Food is the best source of vitamin A because high-dose supplements containing 4–10 times the RNI can cause birth defects and health problems.

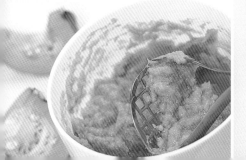

VITAMINS – FAT-SOLUBLE
VITAMIN D

REFERENCE NUTRIENT INTAKE
No RNI because vitamin D can be made in the skin. Except men and women 65+ years: 10 mcg/day. Pregnancy and lactation 10 mcg/day.

FOOD SOURCES	mcg per 100 g
Cod liver oil	210
Kippers, baked	25
Salmon, red, canned in brine	23
Herring, grilled	16.1
Pilchards, canned in tomato sauce	14
Sardines, grilled	12.3
Trout, grilled	11
Salmon, grilled	9.6
Smoked mackerel	8
Low-fat spread and margarines	8
Mackerel, grilled	5.4
Egg yolk	4.9
Sardines, canned in brine	4.6
Tuna, canned in brine	4.0
Evaporated milk	4.0
Fortified breakfast cereals	2.7
Scrambled egg with milk	1.9
Eggs, whole	1.8
Butter	0.8
Beef, lamb, pork, chicken	0.3–0.8
Cheddar cheese	0.3
Yoghurt, whole milk, plain	0.04
Milk, whole	0.03
White fish	Traces
Crustaceans/molluscs	Traces

People with dark skin require less vitamin D than those with fairer skin. Sunscreens with factor 8 or higher actually prohibit the synthesis of vitamin D, but most people get enough sunshine to compensate. Smoke, pollution, window glass and clothing can block sunlight and therefore reduce vitamin D synthesis.

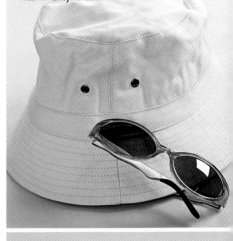

We don't rely on our diet for vitamin D because most of us make enough in our bodies after being in the sun. However, eating sardines is a delicious way to incorporate small amounts of this vitamin and other essential nutrients into our diet.

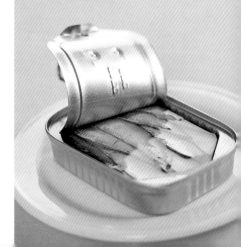

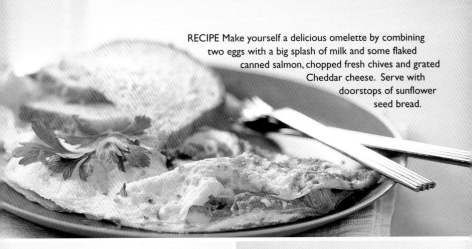

RECIPE Make yourself a delicious omelette by combining two eggs with a big splash of milk and some flaked canned salmon, chopped fresh chives and grated Cheddar cheese. Serve with doorstops of sunflower seed bread.

VITAMIN D is a fat-soluble vitamin. It is known as the sunshine vitamin because it can be made in the skin when the skin is exposed to ultraviolet light. In summer, two hours of sunlight each week is sufficient to maintain adequate levels. Once made, vitamin D is stored in the body for use over the winter, so most people do not have to rely on diet. It is needed for calcium and phosphorus absorption and healthy bones and teeth.

Children need more vitamin D than adults. Without it their bones and teeth will not develop and harden. Adequate sunshine and eating plenty of dairy products regularly throughout life will help keep bones strong.

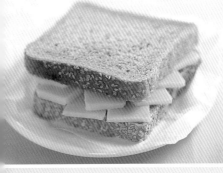

Full-fat milk contains some vitamin D, although skimmed milk contains only traces. Fortified milks are sometimes available, which have added vitamin D.

DEFICIENCY Some people who don't get enough sunlight or vitamin D in their diet are at risk of developing osteomalacia – a condition causing the bones to become soft and easily broken. For more information see page 62. For children, prolonged deficiency may result in rickets, a bone disorder characterised by soft bones, bow legs and curvature of the spine. Vitamin D supplements are advisable for people at risk of osteomalacia.

TOXICITY Too much vitamin D from fortified foods and supplements (more than 50 mcg a day) can be toxic. Effects include sore eyes, itchy skin, vomiting, kidney and heart damage.

VITAMINS – FAT-SOLUBLE

VITAMIN E

SAFE INTAKE:
Men: above 4 mg/day.
Women: above 3 mg/day.

FOOD SOURCES	mg per 100 g
Wheat germ oil	137
Sunflower oil	49.2
Safflower oil	40.7
Sunflower seeds	37.8
Palm oil	33.1
Polyunsaturated margarine	32.6
Hazelnuts	25
Almonds	24
Tomatoes, sun-dried	24
Rapeseed oil	22.2
Wheat germ	22
Mayonnaise	19
Soya oil	16.1
Peanut oil	15.2
Pine nuts	13.6
Salad cream	10.6
Peanuts	10.1
Brazil nuts	7.2
Low-fat spread	6.3
Peanut butter	5
Bombay mix	4.7
Tomatoes, grilled	4
Walnuts	3.8
Pesto sauce	3.8
Avocado	3.2
Sesame seeds	2.5
Butter	2.0
Spinach	1.7
Salmon, pink, canned in brine	1.5
Eggs, raw, boiled or poached	1.1
Broccoli, boiled	1.1
Cheese, Parmesan	0.7

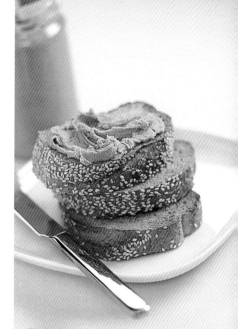

Thick slices of wholegrain bread topped with peanut butter is a great lunch to have to help your vitamin E intake.

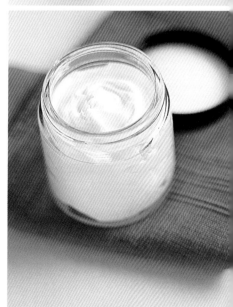

Applied topically in the form of vitamin E cream, the vitamin is absorbed through the skin and promotes wound healing.

Vitamin E is destroyed by heat and exposure to light. Although it's relatively stable at normal cooking temperatures, the high temperatures used in deep-frying, and the repeated heating of the oil, tend to destroy most of the vitamin E. The best way to get this vitamin from oils is in salad dressings.

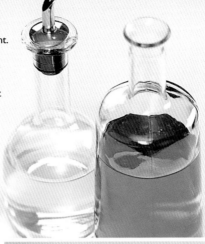

There are eight naturally occurring forms of vitamin E, the most common being alpha-tocopherol. Include plenty of the good sources, such as nuts, plant oils, and wheat germ in your diet.

VITAMIN E is a fat-soluble vitamin and a very powerful antioxidant that neutralises free radical compounds before they can damage cell membranes. It helps protect us from the damage caused by pollution and heavy metals. It is essential for healing, prevention of scarring, and healthy red blood cells and nerves. Deficiency is relatively rare because it is found in many foods.

RECIPE Cook pasta and toss with a kind of pesto made using fresh rocket, almonds, grated Parmesan cheese and oil.

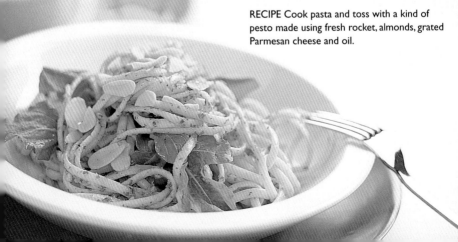

VITAMINS – FAT-SOLUBLE

VITAMIN K

SAFE INTAKE
Adults 1 mcg per kg body weight/day.

FOOD SOURCES	mcg per 100 g*
Spinach	240
Lettuce	200
Soya beans	190
Cauliflower	150
Cabbage	100
Broccoli	100
Wheat bran	80
Wheat germ	37
Green beans	22
Asparagus	21
Oats	20
Potatoes	20
Peas	19
Strawberries	13
Pork	11
Beef mince	7
Milk, full cream	5
Milk, skimmed	4

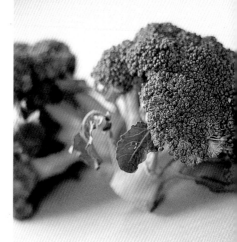

To retain the vitamins in your vegetables, don't cook them too long, but just until they are tender. To prevent vitamin K deficiency, eat plenty of the vegetables listed, including delicious broccoli.

Vitamin K is probably best known for its role in promoting blood clotting to stop bleeding. Because of this, the vitamin is often referred to as the band-aid vitamin.

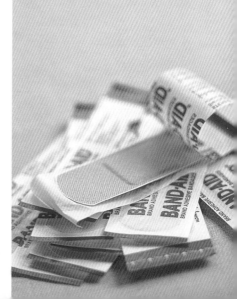

*Australian values.

Eating bio yoghurts (containing acidophilus bacteria) will help you maintain your levels of intestinal bacteria and therefore ensure you make vitamin K in your body. This is particularly useful if you are taking a course of antibiotics, some of which inhibit absorption of the vitamin.

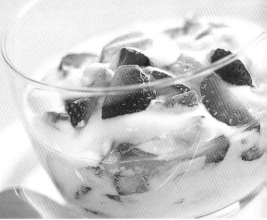

RECIPE Stir-fry sliced pork fillet with broccoli florets, sliced mushrooms, shelled peas, sliced beans, roughly chopped spinach and a little soy sauce and honey.

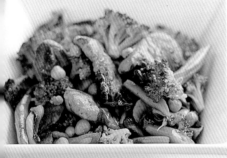

VITAMIN K

VITAMIN K is a fat-soluble vitamin available in a limited number of foods and also made in the body by bacteria which live in our intestinal tract. Babies are given an injection of vitamin K at birth because the infant gut is free of bacteria and breast milk does not contain much of the vitamin. Vitamin K promotes blood clotting and is required for bone mineralisation and kidney function.

Breakfast is a good time to include vitamin K in your diet with plenty of oats, wheat bran, wheat germ and milk.

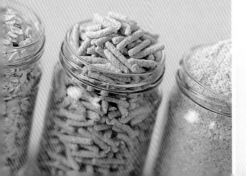

DEFICIENCY This is very rare in healthy people but can result from long-term antibiotic use. Newborn babies are at risk, as explained above, and are therefore injected with the vitamin. Signs of deficiency are easy bruising, and uncontrolled bleeding after injury and surgery.

TOXICITY It is hard to get too much vitamin K from foods, but high doses of supplements containing vitamin K can be dangerous, especially if you are taking anticoagulant drugs. Large doses may also cause flushing and sweating.

ESSENTIAL FATTY ACIDS

No RNI. Suggest approximately 1 per cent of
total energy intake.

SOURCES OF OMEGA-3 FATTY ACIDS

Anchovies, canned, fresh

Canola oil

Cod liver oil

Egg yolk (chicken and duck)

Flaxseed oil

Hazelnuts

Mackerel, canned, fresh

Oysters

Pecans

Prawns

Salmon (pink and red), canned, fresh

Sardines, canned, fresh

Soya bean oil

Squid

Sunflower oil

Tuna, fresh

Vegetables, green leafy

Walnuts

SOURCES OF OMEGA-6 FATTY ACIDS

Canola oil

Corn oil

Dairy and oil spreads

Evening primrose oil

Flaxseed oil

Nuts

Olive oil

Safflower oil

Soya beans

Sunflower oil

If enough omega-3 fatty acids are consumed
in the diet, other important fatty acids can
be synthesised in the body. Oily fish with dark
flesh, such as mackerel, tuna, salmon and
sardines, are the most concentrated source
of omega-3 fatty acids. Aim for two or more
portions of fish every week, one of which
should be an oily fish.

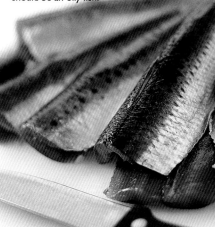

Like other polyunsaturated fats, essential
fatty acids may help control blood cholesterol
levels and reduce the risk of heart disease
when eaten in place of saturated fats in
a low-fat diet.

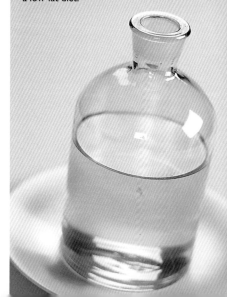

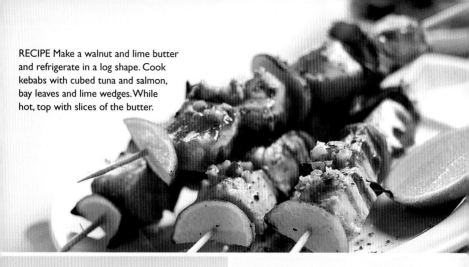

RECIPE Make a walnut and lime butter and refrigerate in a log shape. Cook kebabs with cubed tuna and salmon, bay leaves and lime wedges. While hot, top with slices of the butter.

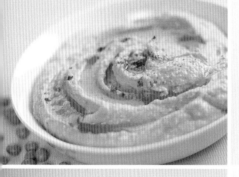

Essential fatty acids must be supplied by the diet. If fish is not your thing, then walnuts, pecans, soya beans and tahini are good sources. Canned soya beans make a tasty houmous.

ESSENTIAL FATTY ACIDS are

fatty acids that can't be made in the body and must be consumed in the diet. Linoleic acid (omega-6) and alpha-linolenic acid (omega-3) are the essential fatty acids and are important for growth, healthy skin and the proper function of eyes and nerves. Linoleic acid and alpha-linolenic acid can be used by the body to make other types of fatty acids.

Cold-pressed vegetable oils, especially sunflower, corn, soya bean, sesame and safflower, are high in omega-6 fatty acids. A balance of both omega-3 and omega-6 is vital and this can be achieved by a mixture of flaxseed oil with the above oils. Canola oil has the best ratio of both omega-3 and omega-6 fatty acids, and soya and walnut oil also contain a mix of both.

DEFICIENCY If essential fatty acids aren't consumed in sufficient amounts, a deficiency results. Symptoms include scaly, dry skin, poor healing of wounds, liver problems, growth failure in infants and impaired vision and hearing.

PROTECTION Although omega-3 fatty acids do not affect cholesterol levels in the blood, they do reduce the tendency for the blood to clot, thereby reducing the risk of heart disease.

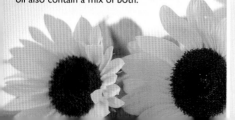

VITAMINS — WATER-SOLUBLE

VITAMIN B1 (THIAMIN)

REFERENCE NUTRIENT INTAKE
Women: 0.8 mg/day (Pregnancy: 0.9 mg/day.
Lactation: 1.0 mg/day). Men 19–50 years: 1.0 mg/day.
Men 51+ years: 0.9 mg/day.

FOOD SOURCES	mg per 100 g
Quorn myco-protein	37
Meat extract	9.7
Yeast extract	4.1
Wheat germ	2
Fortified breakfast cereals	1.03–1.8
Sunflower seeds	1.6
Pork fillet, lean, grilled	1.6
Bacon, back, grilled	1.2
Gammon rashers, grilled	1.2
Peanuts, plain	1.1
Malted milk powder	1.0
Tahini	0.9
Wheat bran	0.9
Sesame seeds	0.9
Ham, lean	0.8
Soya flour	0.8
Peas, boiled	0.7
Pine nuts	0.7
Pistachio nuts, roasted and salted	0.7
Cashew nuts	0.7
Liver, chicken and calf, fried	0.6
Wheat germ	0.5
Kidney, lamb	0.3
Wholemeal bread	0.3
Pasta, wholemeal, boiled	0.2
Kidney beans, canned	0.2
Red split lentils, boiled	0.2
Rice, brown, boiled	0.1
Soya beans, boiled	0.1

RECIPE Stir-fry strips of pork fillet with Chinese leaf, roasted peanuts and soya beans in a little peanut oil. Add soya sauce or oyster sauce. Serve with brown or wild rice timbales.

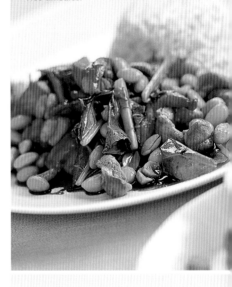

Absorption of thiamin is increased in the presence of allinin, a substance which naturally occurs in garlic and onions.

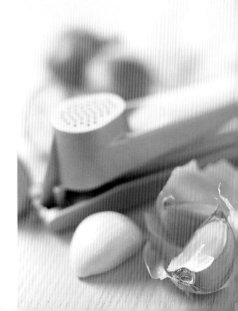

Thiamin occurs in limited quantities in most foods but is available in large quantities in pork and offal.

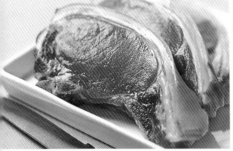

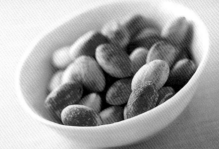

Many nuts, as well as sunflower seeds, will assist in adding thiamin to your diet. However, foods containing sulphur dioxide, such as wine and dried fruits, and sulphite, used in the making of sausages and bacon, can inhibit thiamin absorption.

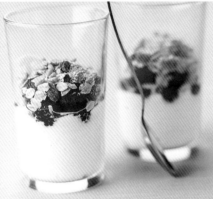

RECIPE For breakfast, layer in a glass some yoghurt, fresh fruit, muesli, oat bran, wheat germ, sunflower and sesame seeds.

VITAMIN B1 (THIAMIN) is a water-soluble vitamin. It is essential for the nervous system and DNA synthesis. Along with other B vitamins, it is needed by the body to produce energy from the nutrients carbohydrate, protein and fat. It is also necessary for growth in childhood and fertility in adults.

Thiamin is found in the germ and bran of wheat and the husk of rice, so consumption of wholegrain bread will provide thiamin in the diet.

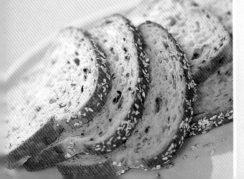

DEFICIENCY Thiamin deficiency is rare but can occur in chronic alcoholics. Extreme deficiency results in the disease beri-beri. Early deficiency symptoms include nausea, muscle fatigue, cramps, depression, irritability and poor coordination. Supplements with relatively large doses of thiamin (50 mg) are marketed for stress relief or an energy boost, but, unless a person has a deficiency, these won't help relieve stress or tiredness. Thiamin absorption is inhibited by an enzyme (thiaminase) present in raw fish and shellfish. Thiamin levels can also be depleted during food preparation, cooking or storage because thiamin is sensitive to heat and oxygen.

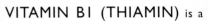

VITAMINS – WATER-SOLUBLE

VITAMIN B2 (RIBOFLAVIN)

REFERENCE NUTRIENT INTAKE
Women: 1.1 mg/day. (Pregnancy: 1.4 mg/day
Lactation: 1.6 mg/day).
Men: 1.3 mg/day.

FOOD SOURCES	mg per 100 g
Yeast extract	11.9
Meat extract	8.5
Liver, lamb, fried	5.7
Kidney, pig, fried	3.7
Liver, chicken, fried	2.7
Fortified breakfast cereals	1.0–2.2
Malted milk powder	1.3
Pâté, liver	1.2
Almonds	0.8
Wheat germ	0.8
Goat's milk soft cheese	0.6
Muesli, Swiss-style	0.7
Hard cheese	0.4–0.5
Egg yolk	0.5
Goose or duck, roasted	0.5
Smoked mackerel	0.5
Tomato-based pasta sauce	0.5
Chocolate, milk	0.5
Tempeh	0.5
Cheese, brie	0.4
Cheese, stilton	0.4
Evaporated milk	0.4
Fromage frais, plain	0.4
Wheat bran	0.4
Eggs, boiled	0.4
Mushrooms, raw	0.3
Pilchards or sardines, canned, in tomato sauce	0.3
Ham hock	0.2
Split peas, boiled	0.06
Kale, boiled	0.06
Spinach, boiled	0.05

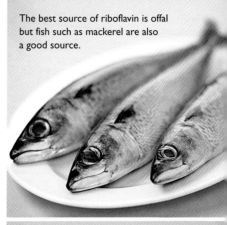

The best source of riboflavin is offal but fish such as mackerel are also a good source.

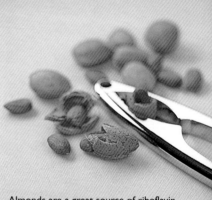

Almonds are a great source of riboflavin. They are a simple snack and easy to add to muesli, salads and stir-fries.

Top up your riboflavin intake first thing in the morning. A breakfast of muesli, a hard-boiled egg and toast with yeast extract is ideal.

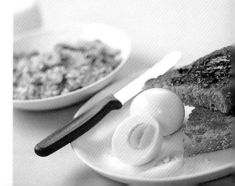

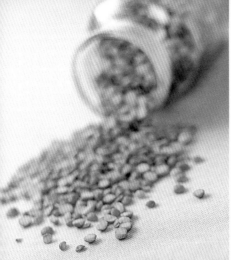

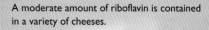

A moderate amount of riboflavin is contained in a variety of cheeses.

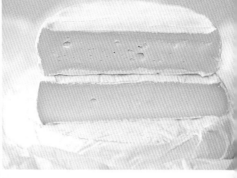

Keep up your riboflavin levels by regularly eating foods containing riboflavin. A simple way of adding a small amount of riboflavin to your diet is to make a delicious split pea soup, using ham hock for flavour. Riboflavin forms part of enzymes which are involved in energy metabolism so you may need more when you are using a lot of energy.

RECIPE Whip up mini mushroom frittatas. Whisk together three eggs, add a generous splash of milk and some chopped fresh flat-leaf parsley and grated Parmesan. Fry some sliced mushrooms and spring onions in butter and add to the eggs. Bake in muffin tins.

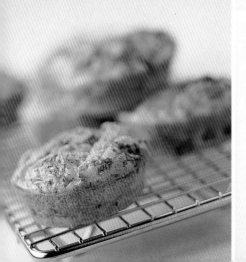

VITAMIN B2 (RIBOFLAVIN) is a

water-soluble vitamin essential for producing energy from carbohydrate, protein and fat. It is necessary for healthy skin, hair and nails, and good vision. It is involved in converting other vitamins (K, B3, B6 and folate) into their active forms in the body. Unlike many vitamins, riboflavin is stable in the presence of heat and acid, but is destroyed by alkali and light.

DEFICIENCY Riboflavin deficiency usually occurs in conjunction with deficiencies in other B vitamins. Deficiency signs are quite obvious, the most common being cracks in the sides of the mouth, a red, sore tongue, or a feeling you have sand in your eyes, which can also be watery or bloodshot. Skin problems are also a sign, especially scaly, flaky dermatitis around the nose and ears. As with thiamin, riboflavin supplements are promoted for an energy boost, but they are not likely to produce any benefits unless a person is truly deficient. Improving your diet gives you more health benefits.

VITAMIN B3 (NIACIN)

REFERENCE NUTRIENT INTAKE

Women 19–50 years: 13 mg NE[+]/day. Women 51+ years: 12 mg NE/day. (Lactation: 15 mg NE/day.) Men 19–50 years: 17 mg NE/day. Men 51+ years: 16 mg NE/day. ([+] NE see page 10.)

FOOD SOURCES	mg per 100 g
Yeast extract	73
Wheat bran	32.6
Liver, lamb, fried	24.8
Tuna, canned in oil	21.1
Fortified breakfast cereals	10–21
Turkey, light meat, roasted	19.7
Peanut butter	19
Liver, calf, fried	19.4
Peanuts, plain	19.3
Chicken, light meat, roasted	18.1
Malted milk powder	17.4
Liver, chicken, fried	17.3
Nuts, mixed	14.8
Mackerel, smoked	13
Beef, fillet, lean, grilled	12.9
Salmon, grilled	12.2
Bacon, back, grilled	11
Sesame seeds	10.4
Salmon, pink, canned in brine	10.3
Tahini	9.2
Sunflower seeds	9.1
Anchovy, canned in oil	8.5
Trout, rainbow, grilled	8.2
Almonds	6.5
Cashew nuts, roasted, salted	6.5
Cheese, Cheddar	6.1
Wholemeal bread	5.9
Eggs, boiled or raw	3.8
Pasta, wholemeal, boiled	2.3
Rice, brown, boiled	1.9
Potatoes, baked	1.1
Milk, whole	0.8

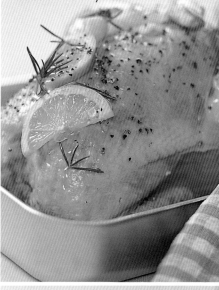

Eating foods such as chicken, fish and nuts, which contain tryptophan, will ensure higher levels of niacin because tryptophan converts to niacin in the body.

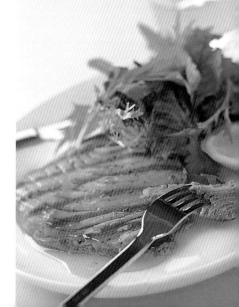

Tuna, trout, salmon, halibut, mackerel and swordfish all contain generous quantities of niacin.

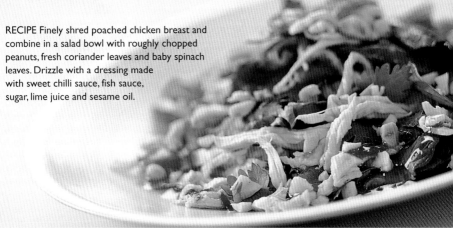

RECIPE Finely shred poached chicken breast and combine in a salad bowl with roughly chopped peanuts, fresh coriander leaves and baby spinach leaves. Drizzle with a dressing made with sweet chilli sauce, fish sauce, sugar, lime juice and sesame oil.

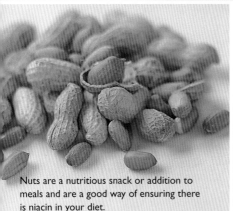

Nuts are a nutritious snack or addition to meals and are a good way of ensuring there is niacin in your diet.

VITAMIN B3 (NIACIN) is an extremely stable water-soluble vitamin and isn't really affected by light, heat, acid, alkali or air. It can be made in the body through the conversion of the amino acid tryptophan. Niacin is important for the production of energy from carbohydrate, protein and fat. It is necessary for healthy skin, tongue and digestive tissues, as well as for normal mental functioning.

Lean white meat from turkey, chicken and veal are higher in niacin than the fattier darker cuts.

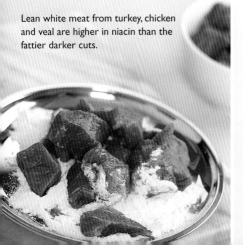

DEFICIENCY Severe deficiency causes pellagra. It is rare in western countries but occurs in countries with food shortages and diets low in protein. A lack of niacin may lead to minor skin problems, weakness, general fatigue and loss of appetite.

TOXICITY If you buy niacin supplements, make sure you buy the nicotinamide form normally sold in the UK. Niacin in the form of nicotinic acid should only be taken on medical advice. Often prescribed to help decrease cholesterol and triglyceride levels, nicotinic acid has the side effect of relaxing blood vessels, causing flushing, red skin rash, high blood sugar levels, itching and even fainting.

VITAMIN B5
(PANTOTHENIC ACID)

No RNI. Intakes of 3–7 mg/day are considered adequate.

FOOD SOURCES	mg per 100 g
Dried yeast	11
Liver, lamb, fried	8.0
Broad beans, canned	6.7
Liver, chicken, fried	5.9
Egg yolk, raw	4.6
Kidney, lamb, fried	4.6
Liver, calf, fried	4.1
Pork fillet, lean, grilled	2.2
Peanuts, plain	2.7
Wheat bran	2.4
Sesame seeds	2.1
Mushrooms, raw	2.0
Salmon, steamed	1.8
Pecan nuts	1.7
Peanut butter	1.7
Soya flour	1.6
Trout, rainbow, grilled	1.6
Chicken breast, grilled, no skin	1.6
Walnuts	1.6
Hazelnuts	1.5
Duck, roast	1.5
Eggs, boiled or poached	1.3
Avocado	1.1
Cashew nuts	1.1
Ham, lean	1.0
Lobster, boiled	1.0
Dried dates	0.8
Dried apricots	0.7
Wholemeal bread	0.6
Cheese, Danish, blue	0.5
Yoghurt, whole, plain	0.5

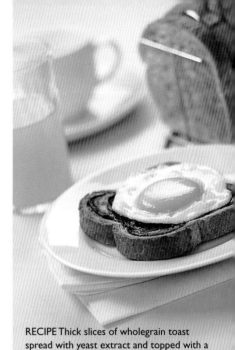

RECIPE Thick slices of wholegrain toast spread with yeast extract and topped with a poached or fried egg.

Pantothenic acid is particularly abundant in animal products including meat, offal, dairy products and eggs. Foods containing moulds, such as mould-ripened cheeses and yoghurts, and yeasts are high in vitamin B5.

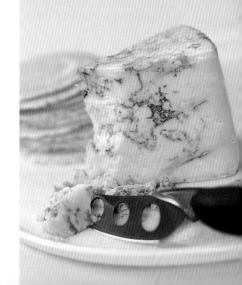

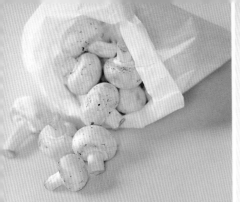

All mushrooms contain a generous amount of vitamin B5, but frying them will reduce the vitamins so it is better to eat them raw.

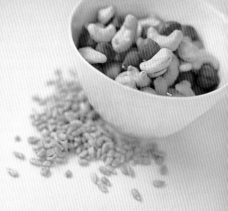

Eating a variety of nuts and seeds is an easy way to top up your B5 intake.

RECIPE Fresh mushroom caps drizzled with melted parsley butter and finished with crumbled blue cheese, then sprinkled with sesame seeds and grilled.

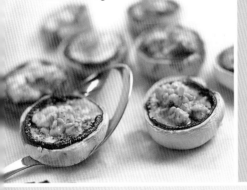

VITAMIN B5 (PANTOTHENIC ACID) is a water-soluble vitamin required for the reactions involved in protein, fat and carbohydrate metabolism. It is needed for fatty acid, cholesterol and steroid hormone synthesis. This vitamin occurs in a wide variety of foods, so deficiency is rare but may be seen with other B vitamin deficiencies, resulting from chronic alcoholism or malnutrition.

Vitamin B5 is depleted through processing and when foods are cooked with acids (vinegars, citrus) and alkali (baking soda). Dry heat cooking methods (frying, grilling) are more damaging to the vitamin than moist heat methods such as stewing and poaching.

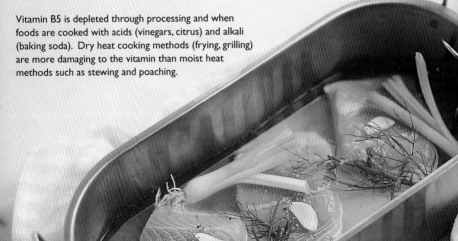

VITAMINS – WATER-SOLUBLE
VITAMIN B6 (PYRIDOXINE)

REFERENCE NUTRIENT INTAKE
Women: 1.2 mg/day.
Men: 1.4 mg/day.

FOOD SOURCES	mg per 100 g
Wheat germ	3.3
Fortified breakfast cereals	0.6–2.7
Dried yeast	2.0
Tempeh	1.9
Yeast extract	1.6
Muesli, swiss-style	1.6
Wheat bran	1.4
Liver, calf, fried	0.9
Salmon, steamed or grilled	0.83
Potato crisps	0.8
Sesame seeds	0.8
Pork fillet, lean, grilled	0.7
Walnuts	0.7
Beef, fillet, lean, grilled	0.61
Chicken breast, grilled, no skin	0.6
Hazelnuts	0.6
Peanuts, plain	0.6
Liver, chicken, fried	0.55
Tuna, canned	0.5
Smoked mackerel	0.5
Red snapper, fried	0.5
Kidney, lamb, fried	0.48
Soya flour	0.46
Haddock, grilled	0.4
Halibut, poached	0.4
Garlic	0.38
Avocado	0.36
Bananas	0.29
Wholemeal bread	0.12

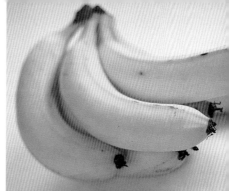

Vitamin B6 is found in a wide variety of plant and animal foods and is added to some breakfast cereals. Boost your levels by adding bananas to your daily diet.

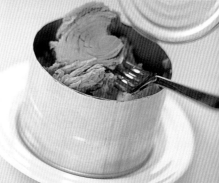

Oily fish are high in vitamin B6. A serving of tuna, salmon or mackerel will provide most of your daily requirement of this vitamin.

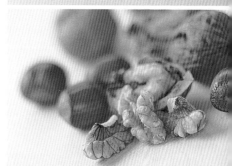

Snacking on unsalted mixed nuts is a good way to get your daily intake of vitamin B6. Eating a cupful of mixed nuts will give you enough B6 for one day.

RECIPE Make a breakfast milkshake that has lots of vitamin B6. Blend soya milk, yoghurt, banana, hazelnuts, wheat germ and maple syrup. Team it with a couple of slices of toasted wholegrain bread topped with sliced tomato and avocado, a drizzle of lime juice and plenty of cracked pepper.

Sashimi salmon is a great way to get B6 into your diet. Thinly slice top-quality boneless salmon fillets and serve with a little soy sauce and wasabi.

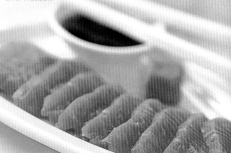

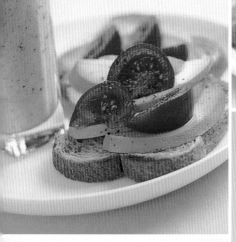

VITAMIN B6 (PYRIDOXINE) is a water-soluble vitamin that is essential for releasing energy from amino acids (protein) and for the metabolism of fat and carbohydrate. It is also required for the normal functioning of the nervous system, as well as the formation of haemoglobin and white cells, and therefore for the immune system.

RECIPE Make wholemeal banana muffins, adding wheat bran and chopped walnuts to the mixture.

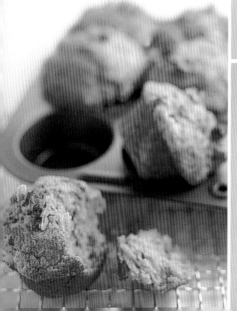

DEFICIENCY A deficiency can result from chronic alcoholism and malnutrition. Symptoms mainly include depression, headaches, confusion, numbness and tingling in the hands and feet, anaemia, skin lesions, decreased immunity and poor growth.

CAUTION Regularly taking high doses of vitamin B6 (more than 50–100 mg/day) should be avoided because it may cause nerve damage. Make sure you check the label of B6 supplements because some contain high doses.

VITAMINS — WATER-SOLUBLE
VITAMIN B12 (COBALAMIN)

REFERENCE NUTRIENT INTAKE
Women and men: 1.5 mcg/day.
Lactation: 2.0 mcg/day.

FOOD SOURCES	mcg per 100 grams
Clams, cooked	99
Liver, lamb	83
Liver, calf, fried	58
Kidney, lamb, fried	54
Cockles, boiled	47
Liver, chicken, fried	45
Winkles, boiled	36
Mussels, boiled	22
Pâté, smoked mackerel	18
Oysters, raw	17
Sardines, canned in oil	15
Kippers, grilled	12
Sardines, grilled	12
Anchovies, canned in oil	11
Kippers, baked	11
Scallops, steamed	9
Pâté, liver	8
Egg yolk	6.9
Salmon, steamed	6
Heart, lamb, roasted	6
Tuna, canned in oil	5.0
Trout, rainbow, grilled	5.0
Lamb, lean, roasted	3.0
Beef, lean, roasted	3.0
Salmon, smoked	3.0
Cheese, Emmental	2.0
Fortified breakfast cereals	1.0–2.2
Cheese, Edam	2.1
Cheese, Cheddar	1.1
Eggs, whole, boiled	1.1
Cheese, feta	1.1
Milk, whole	0.4

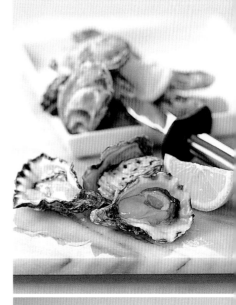

Seafood and fish, especially clams, oysters, sardines and mussels, are a good way to get vitamin B12 and other vital nutrients.

RECIPE Steam clams in a little white wine, chopped tomato, onion and garlic. Discard any that do not open. Sprinkle with a little crumbled feta and chopped fresh parsley.

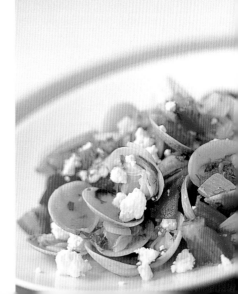

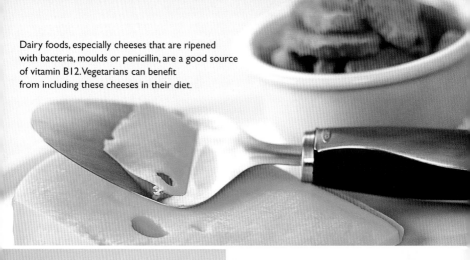

Dairy foods, especially cheeses that are ripened with bacteria, moulds or penicillin, are a good source of vitamin B12. Vegetarians can benefit from including these cheeses in their diet.

Vitamin B12 is widely available in animal foods (beef, lamb, chicken), especially liver and other organ meats, which are particularly rich sources of many vitamins.

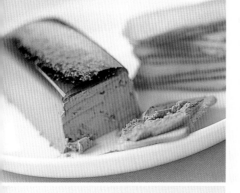

VITAMIN B12 (COBALAMIN) is

a water-soluble vitamin that is essential for growth and the production of energy from fatty acids. It is necessary for DNA synthesis and normal nerve functioning. It can be made by bacteria, fungi and algae, but not by plants and animals.

Fresh egg yolks are a good source of this vitamin, so make an eggflip for a snack.

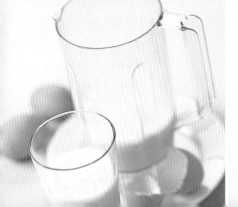

DEFICIENCY The most serious deficiency is pernicious anaemia. Symptoms of deficiency include fatigue, depression, numbness and tingling in the extremities caused by nerve damage, muscle weakness and memory loss. Because plant foods do not contain vitamin B12, strict vegetarians (vegans) may require B12 supplements to meet their requirements. They should also have regular medical checkups as it may take years for deficiency symptoms to appear. People with gastrointestinal disorders are also at risk. Excessive alcohol consumption also hinders absorption. Excess vitamin B12 is readily excreted in urine and there are no known adverse effects from a high intake.

VITAMINS – WATER-SOLUBLE
FOLATE or FOLIC ACID

REFERENCE NUTRIENT INTAKE
Women and men: 200 mcg/day.
(Pregnancy: 300 mcg/day, see also 'Extra needs'
opposite. Lactation: 260 mcg/day.)

FOOD SOURCES	mcg per 100 g
Dried yeast	4000
Liver, chicken, fried	1350
Yeast extract	1150
Meat extract	1050
Soya flour	345
Wheat germ	331
Fortified breakfast cereals	150–330
Liver, lamb, fried	260
Black-eye beans, boiled	210
Sweetcorn, baby, fresh or frozen, boiled	152
Pinto beans, boiled	145
Broccoli, purple sprouting, boiled	140
Muesli, Swiss-style	140
Egg yolk	130
Brussels sprouts, boiled	110
Peanuts	110
Cheese, Camembert	102
Swiss chard, boiled	100
Pâté, liver	99
Sesame seeds	97
Spinach, boiled	90
Cheese, Stilton	77
Hazelnuts	72
Cashew nuts	67
Walnuts	66
Spring greens, boiled	66
Wholemeal rolls	62
Oatmeal	60
Green beans, boiled	57
Lettuce	55
Soya beans, boiled	54
Oranges	31

RECIPE Make the greenest of green salads with cos lettuce, lightly steamed broccoli florets, asparagus, baby spinach, soya beans and avocado. Dress with an orange, soya and walnut oil dressing to accompany a big bowl of chilli con carne.

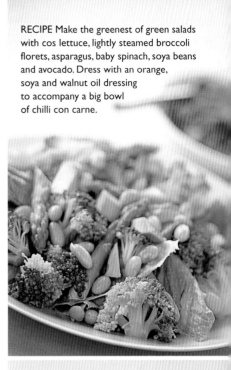

A diet high in beans and pulses will ensure that you have high levels of folic acid. Bean salads are easy to prepare and last for up to a week in the refrigerator in an airtight container. Delicious served hot or cold.

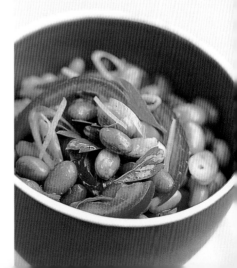

DRIED YEAST is a very rich source of folate. Adding a teaspoonful to a banana and date milkshake with a tablespoon of wheat germ is an easy way to have it.

Green leafy vegetables such as spinach, broccoli and lettuce are an excellent way to obtain folate. However, things such as cooking at high temperatures, light, and lengthy storage at room temperature will destroy it, so remember that eating the vegetables fresh or lightly steamed or stir-fried is best.

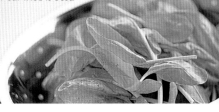

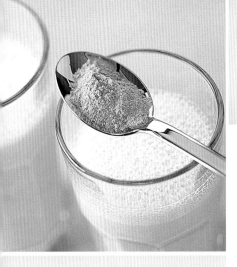

FOLATE or FOLIC ACID is a

vitamin essential for the nervous system and proper functioning of the brain. It is also necessary for growth and reproduction of body cells. It is vital for the healthy development of babies in utero. Folic acid takes its name from the Latin word for foliage or leaf.

RECIPE For a delicious folate-filled vegetable accompaniment, lightly steam purple sprouting broccoli and green beans and top with chopped hazelnuts and sunflower and sesame seeds. Drizzle with lemon-infused butter.

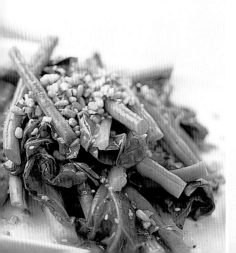

EXTRA NEEDS Though relatively rare, a severe folic acid deficiency can cause a form of anaemia (megaloblastic anaemia), a sore, red tongue, chronic diarrhoea and poor growth (in children). Low levels of folic acid intake have no symptoms but may raise the risk of heart disease and birth defects.

CAUTION Pregnant women are advised to take a 400 mcg folic acid supplement every day until the twelfth week of pregnancy. Getting sufficient folic acid is thought to reduce the risk of the baby being born with neural tube defects.

VITAMINS – WATER-SOLUBLE
VITAMIN C (ASCORBIC ACID)

REFERENCE NUTRIENT INTAKE
Women and men: 40 mg/day.
(Pregnancy: 50 mg/day. Lactation: 70 mg/day.)

FOOD SOURCES	mg per 100 g
Guava	230
Red chillies	225
Blackcurrants	200
Parsley	190
Red peppers (capsicum)	140
Green peppers (capsicum)	120
Spring greens	77
Strawberries	77
Curly kale, boiled	71
Watercress	62
Cabbage, Savoy	62
Brussels sprouts, boiled	60
Papaya (pawpaw)	60
Kiwi	59
Red cabbage, raw	55
Oranges	54
Orange juice, freshly squeezed	48
Broccoli, boiled	44
Tomatoes, grilled	44
Cauliflower	43
Redcurrants	40
Sweetcorn, baby, fresh or frozen, boiled	39
Orange juice, unsweetened	39
Lime juice	38
Nectarines	37
Mango	37
Grapefruit	36

(continued)

RECIPE Char-grill tuna or chicken pieces and top with a salsa made with mango, tomato, red onion, chilli, and red and green peppers. Serve on finely shredded Chinese cabbage, which has been tossed with a little sesame oil, lime juice and fresh parsley.

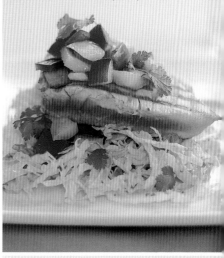

RECIPE A delicious drink made with mixed berries, orange juice, papaya and ice, blended until smooth, will help boost your vitamin C intake.

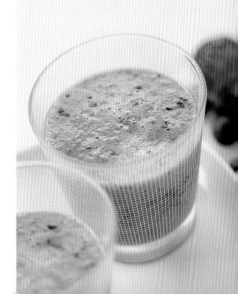

It is easy to obtain your daily vitamin C requirements by eating plenty of fruit and vegetables. The fresher they are, the more vitamins they contain, so try growing your own. Chillies and herbs grow easily.

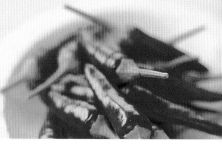

VITAMIN C (ASCORBIC ACID) is a water-soluble vitamin required for the formation of connective tissue such as collagen, necessary for the formation of healthy skin, bones, cartilage and teeth. Vitamin C is also needed for the synthesis of neuro-transmitters, hormones, such as thyroid and sex hormones, and carnitine needed for fatty acid breakdown.

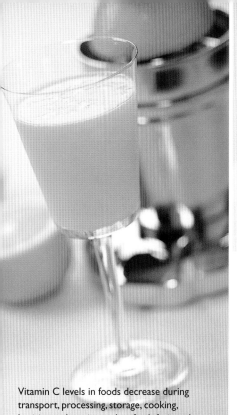

Vitamin C levels in foods decrease during transport, processing, storage, cooking, bruising and cutting, so buy fresh fruit and vegetables regularly. Vitamin C survives longer in citrus fruits than all other fruits and vegetables. Orange juice will retain its vitamin C content for up to two days if kept in an airtight container in the refrigerator.

Vitamin C is the least stable of all the vitamins and is extremely sensitive to oxygen, light, heat, and certain metals including copper and iron. Cooking reduces the vitamin C in foods by about 50 per cent. Microwaving, steaming and stir-frying help preserve vitamin C and are the most suitable cooking methods.

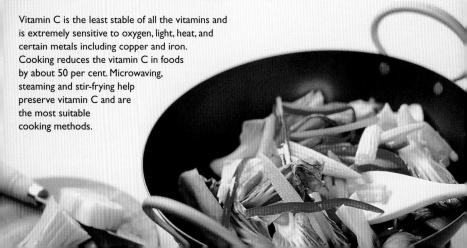

VITAMIN C (ASCORBIC ACID)

FOOD SOURCES (continued)	mg per 100 g
Salad, green	36
Raspberries	32
Red cabbage, boiled	32
Sugar snap peas	32
Grapefruit juice, unsweetened	31
Peaches	31
Tomatoes, cherry	28
Cauliflower, boiled	27
Satsumas	27
Melon, cantaloupe-type	26
Spinach	26
Spring onions	26
Gooseberries	26
Mango juice, canned	25
Liver, chicken, fried	23
Sweet potato, baked	23
Passion fruit	23
Cabbage, chinese	21
Courgette, raw	21
Coleslaw (with mayonnaise)	20
Broad beans, boiled	20
Cabbage, boiled	20
Garlic	17
Bilberries	17
Radish, red	17
Peas, boiled	16
Courgette, boiled	11

RECIPE Lightly steam broccoli, drizzle with lime juice and sesame oil and finish with oyster sauce and slices of fried garlic.

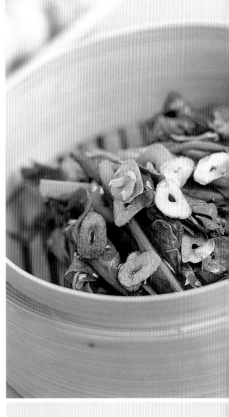

There is a limit to the amount of vitamin C our body tissues absorb at one time so it is recommended that we consume regular, small doses of it throughout the day by eating vitamin C rich foods. Any excess that the body does not use is excreted in urine.

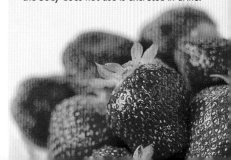

RECIPE Make a delicious sweet couscous by very gently heating 450 ml (1 pint) orange juice, then pouring it over 175 g (6 oz) of couscous. Add 1 cinnamon stick, cover and allow to stand until all the liquid is absorbed. Serve with a freshly prepared fruit salad.

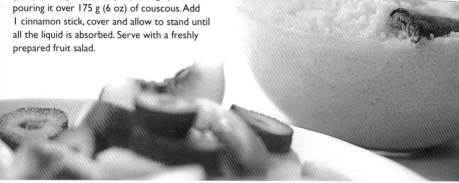

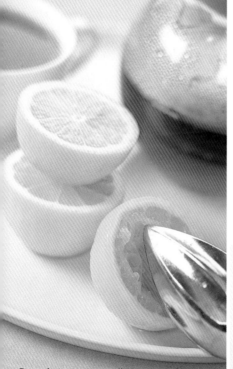

VITAMIN C (ASCORBIC ACID)

acts as an antioxidant to protect the body against damage caused by free radicals and pollutants such as cigarette smoke and air pollution. People who smoke may need to consume up to twice the RNI to maintain their vitamin C levels because their body has to use so much of it to protect the body's tissues from cigarette smoke and chemicals. Vitamin C also promotes healing and iron absorption.

DEFICIENCY Signs are increased susceptibility to infection, loss of appetite, muscle cramps, dry skin, splitting hair, bleeding gums, impaired digestion, anaemia, nosebleeds and bruising. Scurvy can occur in babies fed only cow's milk, in alcoholics and in elderly people with poor diets.

CAUTION More than 1 g a day can cause abdominal cramps, diarrhoea and nausea. More than 3 g a day can interfere with drugs that slow blood clotting, and with tests that monitor blood glucose levels. People with kidney problems or a genetic tendency to store excess iron should not take high doses.

Citrus fruits are an excellent source of vitamin C. Vitamin C stimulates the activity of the immune system and increases the breakdown of histamine, a molecule that causes inflammation. Vitamin C helps protect the body against viruses. For these reasons, it may reduce the severity of cold symptoms.

VITAMINS – WATER-SOLUBLE
BIOTIN

No RNI. Intakes between 10 and 200 mcg/day are considered adequate and safe.

FOOD SOURCES	mcg per 100 g
Liver, chicken, fried	216
Dried yeast	200
Peanuts, roasted, salted	102
Peanut butter	102
Mixed nuts	86
Almonds	64
Plaice, grilled	57
Liver, calf, fried	50
Egg yolk	50
Wheat bran	45
Liver, lamb, fried	33
Wheat germ	25
Soya beans, boiled	25
Eggs, whole	20
Oatmeal	20
Walnuts	19
Muesli, Swiss-style	15
Pâté, liver	14
Cashew nuts, plain	13
Haggis, boiled	12
Pilchards, canned in tomato sauce	11
Brazil nuts	11
Kippers, baked	10
Salmon, pink, canned in brine	9
Salmon, grilled	9
Cheese, Camembert	8
Cheese, hard	3
Milk, semi-skimmed	2
Yoghurt, whole milk, fruit	2

A nut spread instead of butter or margarine on bread will not only add flavour but also increase the biotin and vitamin content of your diet.

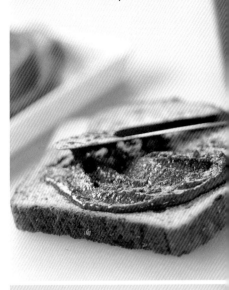

Unlike a lot of other vitamins, biotin is stable to light, heat and acid. Raw egg white contains avidin (a protein that prevents biotin absorption), but avidin is destroyed by cooking egg white.

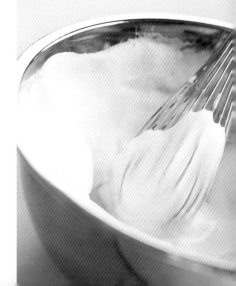

RECIPE Lightly fry thinly sliced lamb's liver in a little oil and butter with chopped onion and pieces of bacon. Thicken with some flour and a little stock, then simmer until you have a rich gravy.

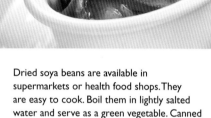

Dried soya beans are available in supermarkets or health food shops. They are easy to cook. Boil them in lightly salted water and serve as a green vegetable. Canned soya beans are also available.

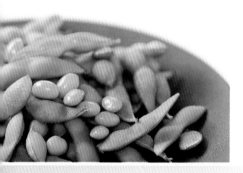

BIOTIN, a member of the B complex group, is required for cell growth and the metabolism of protein, folic acid, B5 and B12. It plays a special role in helping the body to use glucose, as well as promoting healthy hair and nails. Without biotin in the diet, the ability of the body to break down fatty foods is impaired.

RECIPE Oatmeal, wheat bran and nuts all provide biotin in the diet so why not kickstart your day with a bowl of porridge topped with wheat bran, nuts and fruit.

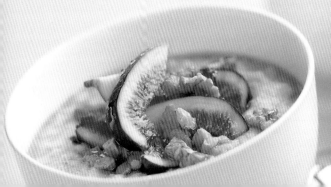

NUTRIENTS – WATER-SOLUBLE
FLAVONOIDS

No RNI. Exact values are difficult to obtain.

FOOD SOURCES

Apricots

Beetroot

Blackberries

Blackcurrants

Blueberries

Broad beans

Broccoli

Buckwheat

Cabbage

Cherries

Cranberries

Endive

Garlic

Grapefruit

Grapes

Green tea

Lemons

Limes

Mandarins

Melon

Mulberries

Onions

Oranges

Papaya (pawpaw)

Parsley

Pecans

Peppers (capsicum)

Plums

Potatoes

Prunes

Radishes

Raspberries

Rosehips

Squash

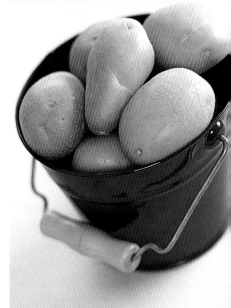

Quercetin is a flavonoid found in citrus fruits, berries, tomatoes and potatoes and may help to reduce histamine production and allergy and inflammatory symptoms.

These powerful antioxidants are found in most fruits and vegetables and this may partly explain why the regular consumption of a wide variety of fresh fruits and vegetables appears to reduce the risk of heart disease and some cancers.

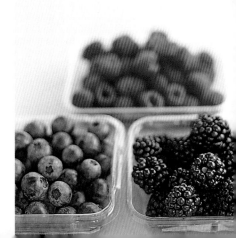

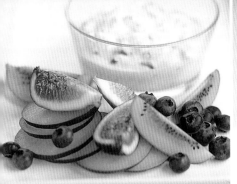

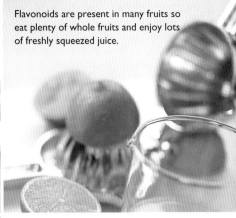

Flavonoids are present in many fruits so eat plenty of whole fruits and enjoy lots of freshly squeezed juice.

RECIPE For a flavonoid boost, serve a home-made berry yoghurt with fresh fruits, including more berries.

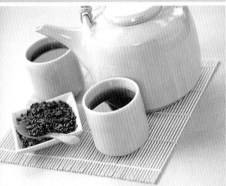

To assist your intake of flavonoids, you can substitute your afternoon cuppa with soothing green tea or replace that beer with a glass of red wine.

FLAVONOIDS are a group of phytochemicals found in all plants. More than 4000 flavonoids have been identified so far. They are antioxidants that can be found in most fruits and vegetables. They are usually found in flowers, and accompany vitamin C in the leaves and stems of brightly coloured fruits, vegetables and plants. They prevent oxidation in the tissues and mop up free radicals. They seem to be more powerful antioxidants than vitamins C, E and selenium.

RECIPE Purée cooked, peeled beetroot, add some garlic and broad beans and mix with a little stock.

FLAVONOIDS are also pigment compounds that give the red and blue colours to blueberries, raspberries and red cabbage, and the pale yellow colour in potatoes, onions and citrus rind. They are richest in the pith and peel of citrus fruit rather than juice, so add these to salads, or juice, in small quantities as they can be quite bitter.

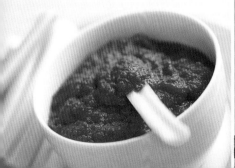

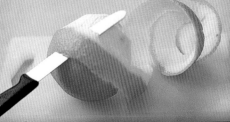

NUTRIENTS – WATER SOLUBLE
INOSITOL

No RNI. Exact values are difficult to obtain,
and it can be made in the body.

FOOD SOURCES

Barley
Black-eye peas
Bread, wholemeal
Cabbage
Chickpeas
Dried yeast
Grapefruit
Lentils
Lettuce
Lima beans
Melon, cantaloupe-type
Oatmeal
Onions
Oranges
Peanut butter
Peanuts, roasted
Peas, green
Pecans
Raisins
Rice bran
Rice, brown
Rice germ
Soya flour
Soya beans
Strawberries
Watermelon
Wheat germ

Lightly cook lentils in a stock with a bay leaf
and clove-studded onion. Season with salt
and pepper and chopped fresh herbs. These
lentils make a perfect accompaniment to
any meal.

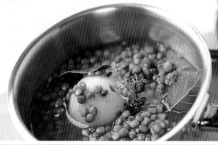

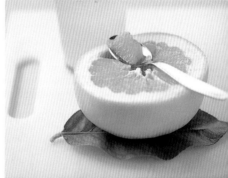

All citrus fruits except lemons, juiced or
eaten in their natural form, provide inositol
in generous quantities.

Lettuce and other foods on the list are all
good sources of inositol as well as other
vitamins and minerals.

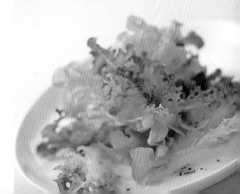

RECIPE Home-made muesli is a good way to combine foods that contain inositol. Mix oatmeal, wheat germ, rice bran, raisins and nuts. Store in an airtight container.

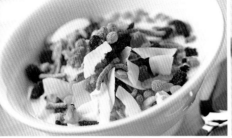

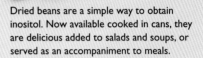

Dried beans are a simple way to obtain inositol. Now available cooked in cans, they are delicious added to salads and soups, or served as an accompaniment to meals.

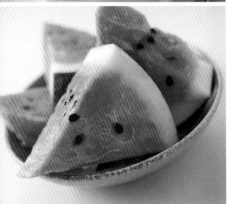

Half a cantaloupe melon, a punnet of strawberries, or a big wedge of watermelon will boost inositol levels.

INOSITOL works in a similar way to choline (see page 57) and, like choline, is not a vitamin because it can be made in the body from glucose. It is a component of the fatty compounds in cell membranes where it plays a role in relaying the messages from hormones and neuro-transmitters to the inside of the cell. It appears to be involved in the metabolism of cholesterol and fat. Inositol combines with choline to make lecithin.

Barley makes a delicious accompaniment to any meal and is as easy to cook as rice. To give it extra flavour, substitute the water with stock or the reserved liquid from rehydrated dried mushrooms.

DEFICIENCY Deficiency is rare and unlikely in healthy people. Inositol can be synthesised from glucose and has not been shown to be essential in the diet as it can be made in the body.

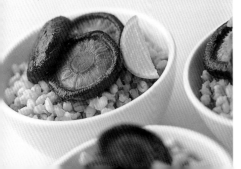

NUTRIENTS – WATER-SOLUBLE
CHOLINE

No RNI because it can be made in the body
to some extent.

FOOD SOURCES

Barley

Beef

Black-eye peas

Black treacle

Brains

Cabbage

Cauliflower

Chickpeas

Dried yeast

Eggs

Egg yolk

Grape juice

Ham

Kidneys, all types

Lentils

Lettuce

Liver, all types

Oatmeal

Peanuts, roasted

Peanut butter

Pork

Potatoes

Rice, brown

Soya beans

Spinach

Split peas

Sweet potatoes

Textured Vegetable Protein (TVP)

Veal

Wheat bran

Wheat germ

Lecithin is the richest source of choline and
is used as a food additive in ice cream,
margarine, chocolate, mayonnaise and baked
goods to keep the oil separating from the
other ingredients (as an emulsifying agent).

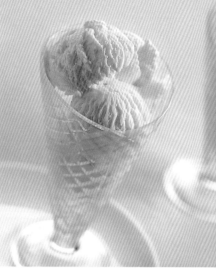

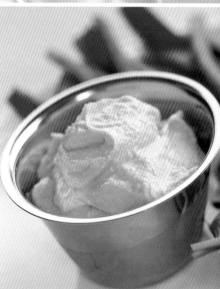

A bowl of houmous served with steamed
green vegetable crudités is a great nutritious
snack when studying – choline is responsible
for a chemical in the brain that aids memory.

RECIPE Whisk together eggs, milk and grated Cheddar. Season with salt and pepper, add finely shredded spinach leaves and chunks of steamed sweet potato. Bake until set.

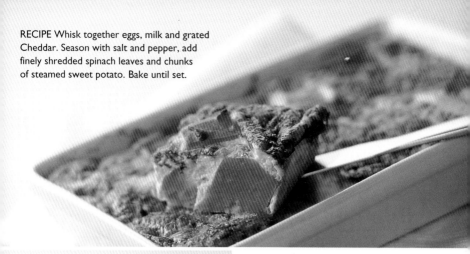

One egg will provide you with roughly enough choline for one day.

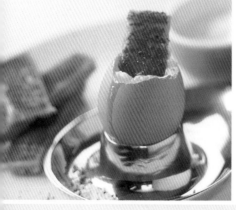

CHOLINE is not classified as a vitamin because it can be made in the body to some extent, but there is evidence that it is essential in the diet during certain stages of life. It is required for the synthesis of the neurotransmitter, acetylcholine, which is involved in nerve and brain functioning and memory. Deficiency is rare but causes liver problems.

A ham and egg sandwich using wholemeal bread will help add some of this essential compound to your diet.

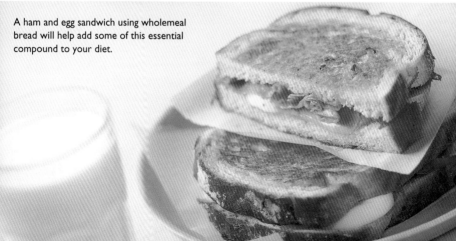

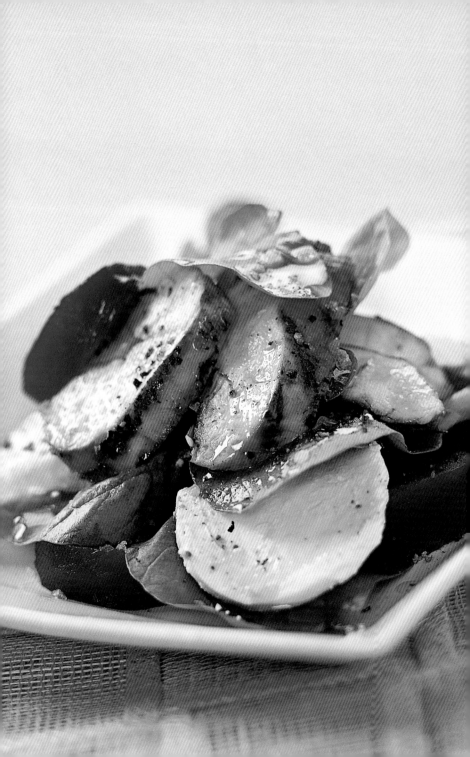

minerals

MINERALS – MAJOR
CALCIUM

REFERENCE NUTRIENT INTAKE
Women and men: 700 mg/day.
(Lactation: 1250 mg/day.)

FOOD SOURCES	mg per 100 g
Cheese, Parmesan	1200
Cheese, Emmental	970
Cheese, Gruyère	950
Cheese, Edam	770
Cheese, Cheddar	720
Tahini	680
Sesame seeds	670
Pesto sauce	560
Cheese, Brie	540
Sardines, canned in brine	540
Tofu, soya bean, steamed	510
Malted milk powder	430
Seaweed, nori, dried	430
Salmon, pink, canned, flesh and bone	300
Carob powder	390
Evaporated milk, whole	290
Almonds	240
Figs, ready-to-eat	230
Chocolate, milk	220
Soya flour	210
Parsley	200
Yoghurt, low fat, plain	190
Spinach	170
Watercress	170
Curly kale, boiled	150
Tortilla chips	150
Greek yoghurt	150
Muffins	140
Hazelnuts	140
Oysters	140
Vanilla ice cream	130

(continued)

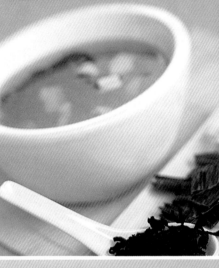

RECIPE Kelp, wakame and nori are varieties of seaweed used in Japanese cooking. To make a quick miso soup, simmer kelp, miso and dashi granules for 10 minutes before adding small cubes of tofu. Sprinkle with strips of roasted seaweed if desired.

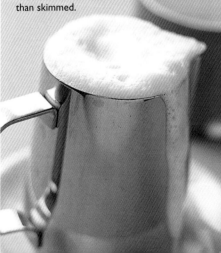

Calcium is most readily absorbed from dairy products because lactose (milk sugar) enhances calcium absorption. If you are lactose intolerant, you may still be able to tolerate 2–3 servings of dairy, consumed in small quantities over a day. Full-cream milk may be easier to digest than skimmed.

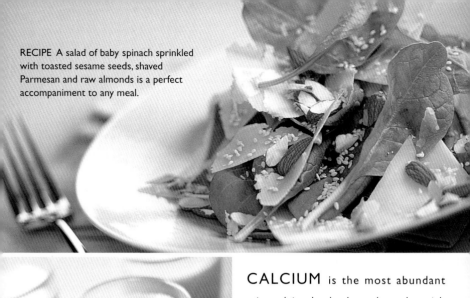

RECIPE A salad of baby spinach sprinkled with toasted sesame seeds, shaved Parmesan and raw almonds is a perfect accompaniment to any meal.

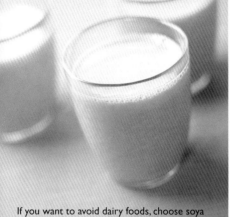

If you want to avoid dairy foods, choose soya milk products fortified with calcium.

CALCIUM is the most abundant mineral in the body and works with phosphorus and other elements to give strength to bones and teeth. Calcium is necessary for blood clotting and the transmission of nerve impulses. It is essential in enzyme regulation, in the secretion of insulin in adults, and in the regulation of muscle function. Vitamin D is required for calcium absorption.

Contrary to popular belief, there is no need for extra calcium during pregnancy. This is because a woman's body becomes more efficient at absorbing calcium during pregnancy. More is recommended during breast-feeding as a precaution. Children and adolescents need to make sure they are getting enough calcium to ensure growth. Cheese is one of the richest sources of calcium. Try Swiss cheeses, such as Emmental.

MINERALS – MAJOR
CALCIUM

FOOD SOURCES (continued)	mg per 100 g
Tempeh	120
Pineapple, dried	120
Wheat germ bread	120
Milk, skimmed or semi-skimmed	120
Milk, whole	115
White bread	110
Broccoli, purple sprouting	110
Prawns, boiled	110
Currant buns	110
Sunflower seeds	110
Cream crackers	110
Scones, wholemeal	110
Cottage cheese, plain	110
Muesli Swiss-style	110
Cream cheese	98
Walnuts	94
Cream, fresh, soured	93
Apricots, dried	92
Fish fingers, cod, grilled	92
Cream, fresh, single	91
Fromage frais, plain	89
Tzatziki	88
Mackerel, canned in tomato sauce	82
Miso	73
Red kidney beans, canned	71
Haricot beans, boiled	65
Sultanas	64
Pecan nuts	61
Eggs, whole, raw or poached	57
Broccoli	56
Oatmeal	55
Sugar snap peas	54
Baked beans, canned in tomato sauce	53
Oranges	47
Chickpeas, boiled	46

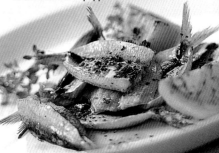

Fresh or canned sardines, if eaten with the bones, are a rich source of calcium. Drizzle with lemon juice and sprinkle with plenty of cracked black pepper.

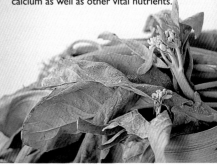

Calcium is required for blood clotting, muscle contraction and nerve function. Although the calcium in spinach and other vegetables isn't as well absorbed as the calcium in dairy foods, it can still provide you with some calcium as well as other vital nutrients.

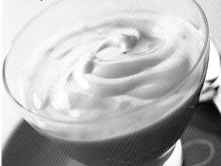

Calcium absorption is enhanced by lactose, the natural sugar present in milk and dairy products, so calcium in dairy products is easily absorbed. A big bowl of yoghurt is an easy calcium-rich snack.

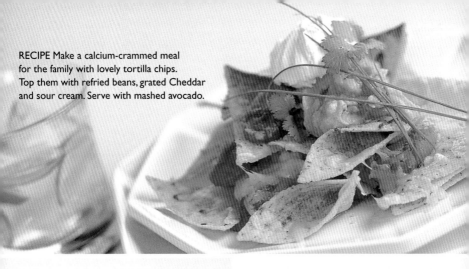

RECIPE Make a calcium-crammed meal for the family with lovely tortilla chips. Top them with refried beans, grated Cheddar and sour cream. Serve with mashed avocado.

Nuts and seeds are a good source of calcium, especially sesame seeds which can be used to coat foods, add flavour to salads, or used as tahini paste as a spread for bread.

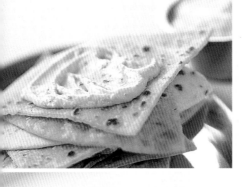

Next time you are baking, try substituting carob powder for cocoa powder to add more calcium to the product.

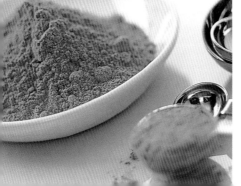

CALCIUM As children, teenagers and young adults, bones not only grow in length and width, they also become more dense as the amount of calcium and other minerals they contain increase. This makes them strong and the stronger they are, the less likely they are to fracture and break. Provided we get enough calcium, bone density will increase until our late 20s or early 30s, when it will reach its peak. From then on, more bone cells are removed than are replaced and because of this, bone gets thinner as we get older. This is a normal part of ageing, but if you have a low peak bone mass, you may lose more bone cells as you age and develop osteoporosis (brittle bone disease) in later life. Oestrogen helps to maintain calcium in the bones, so bone loss is accelerated in women after the menopause. Even though peak bone mass is reached in early life, it is important to maintain an adequate calcium intake as you get older.

DEFICIENCY Signs of calcium deficiency include osteoporosis, osteomalacia, muscle spasms and cramping, heart palpitations, high blood pressure, rickets and joint pain. Most people would not benefit from calcium supplements as it is not difficult to get enough from diet alone.

MINERALS – MAJOR
MAGNESIUM

REFERENCE NUTRIENT INTAKE
Women: 270 mg/day.
(Lactation: 320 mg/day.)
Men: 300 mg/day.

FOOD SOURCES	mg per 100 g
Wheat bran	520
Cocoa powder	520
Seaweed, dried, wakame	470
Brazil nuts	410
Sunflower seeds	390
Tahini	380
Sesame seeds	310
Winkles, boiled	340
Wheat germ	270
Cashew nuts, plain	270
Almonds	270
Pine nuts	270
Dried yeast	230
Peanuts	210
Peanut butter	180
Oat and wheat bran	180
Black treacle	180
Walnuts	160
Yeast extract	160
Hazelnuts	160
Shrimps, boiled	110
Crispbread, rye	100
Mustard, wholegrain	93
Swiss chard, boiled	86
Figs, dried	80
Wholemeal bread	76
Tempeh	70
Apricots, dried	65
Soya beans, boiled	63
Houmous	62
Prawns, boiled	49
Spinach, boiled	34
Tofu	23

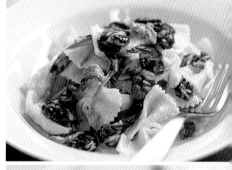

Magnesium is found in green leafy vegetables, so add some wilted spinach to pasta dishes, salads and sandwiches.

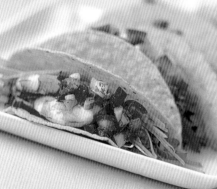

RECIPE Prawn or tofu tacos filled with shredded spinach, tomato, carrot and salsa.

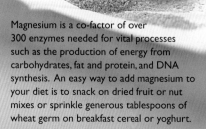

Magnesium is a co-factor of over 300 enzymes needed for vital processes such as the production of energy from carbohydrates, fat and protein, and DNA synthesis. An easy way to add magnesium to your diet is to snack on dried fruit or nut mixes or sprinkle generous tablespoons of wheat germ on breakfast cereal or yoghurt.

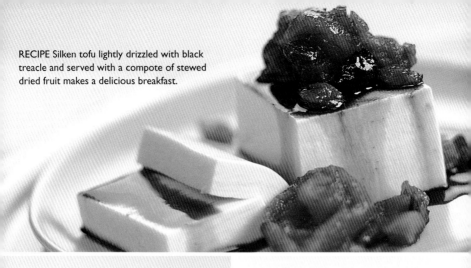

RECIPE Silken tofu lightly drizzled with black treacle and served with a compote of stewed dried fruit makes a delicious breakfast.

Magnesium is involved in regulating calcium balance in the body and is needed for the action of vitamin D and many hormones, so eat plenty of foods containing magnesium.

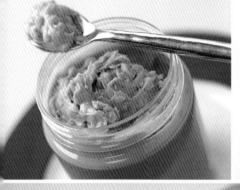

MAGNESIUM, along with calcium and phosphorus, is needed for strong, healthy bones and proper nerve and muscle functioning. It is essential for the action of vitamin D, and hence, calcium absorption, and many hormones. Symptoms of low levels of magnesium in the body are muscle spasms, tremors, cramping, twitching, changes in blood pressure and heartbeat. It is difficult to get too much magnesium as the absorption decreases as intake increases and the kidneys are very efficient at eliminating any excess.

RECIPE Sesame and sunflower seeds are a rich source of magnesium. Combined with crushed almonds, pine nuts and cashews and mixed with ricotta and herbs, they make a delicious filling for veal, chicken or pork, or can be sprinkled on baked mushrooms.

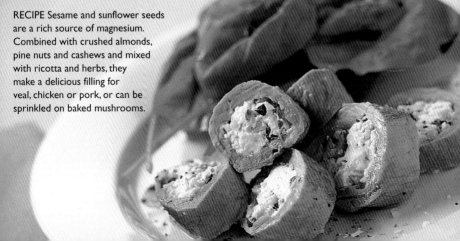

MINERALS – MAJOR
PHOSPHORUS

REFERENCE NUTRIENT INTAKE
Women and men: 550 mg/day.
(Lactation: 990 mg/day.)

FOOD SOURCES	mg per 100 g
Dried yeast	1290
Wheat bran	1200
Wheat germ	1050
Processed cheese, smoked	1030
Yeast extract	950
Pumpkin seeds	850
Cheese spread	790
Sesame seeds	720
Pine nuts	650
Sunflower seeds	640
Cheese, Gruyère	610
Brazil nuts	590
Cheese, Emmental	590
Cashew nuts	560
Almonds	550
Sardines, canned in oil	520
Egg yolk	500
Cheese, Cheddar	490
Pesto sauce	480
Monkfish, grilled	480
Pâté, liver	450
Kipper, baked	430
Kidney, pig, fried	430
Sardines, canned in tomato sauce	420
Liver, calf, fried	380
Walnuts	380
Oatmeal	380
Peanut butter	370
Kidney, lamb, fried	350
Chicken breast, grilled, no skin	310
Cheese, Feta	280
Milk	92

RECIPE Char-grill chicken breast fillets that have been marinated in lemon juice or vinegar, sesame seeds, garlic and kecap manis. Cook until tender, then serve sliced on a rocket, goat's cheese and beetroot salad dressed with olive oil and garlic.

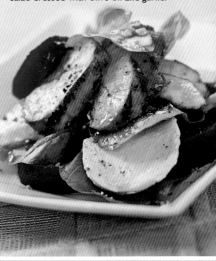

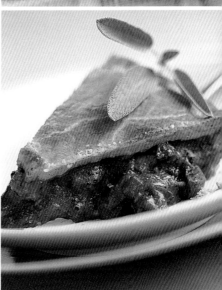

Protein-rich foods are high in phosphorus, with offal containing greater levels than a steak. Steak and kidney pie is a delicious way of sneaking offal into your diet.

RECIPE For a phosphorus-rich vegetarian meal, pan-fry or barbecue mushrooms, top with chunks of marinated feta with a little of its oil and finish with canned spicy Mexican beans.

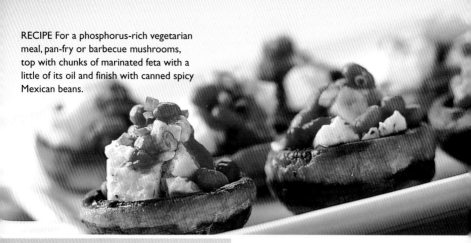

RECIPE Roast unsalted pumpkin seeds in a little honey and black sesame seeds for 15 minutes in a moderate oven. This simple snack is a good way to obtain phosphorus.

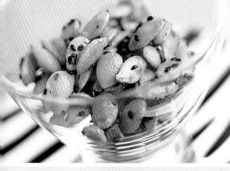

PHOSPHORUS is the second most abundant mineral in the body after calcium. It is present in every cell of the body and has important structural roles. Teamed with calcium, it is necessary for bone strength. Phosphorus is required for almost every chemical reaction in the body and for energy production. Deficiency is rare because it's in a variety of foods – even more than calcium.

Phosphorus is easily absorbed by the body; more easily even than calcium. Some dairy products, including low-fat varieties, contain relatively large amounts of phosphorus.

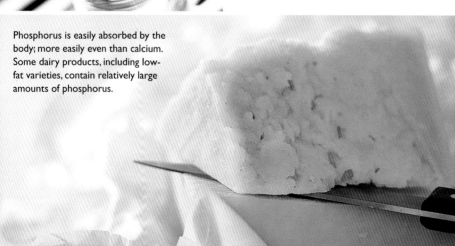

MINERALS – MAJOR
SODIUM

REFERENCE NUTRIENT INTAKE
Women and men: 1600 mg/day

FOOD SOURCES	mg per 100 g
Salt	39300
Bicarbonate of soda	38700
Stock cubes	10300
Soy sauce	7120
Instant gravy granules	6330
Meat extract	4370
Yeast extract	4300
Shrimps, boiled	3840
Miso	3650
Instant soup powder	3440
Bacon, back, grilled	2240
Olives in brine	2000
Ham, gammon, grilled	1930
Salmon, smoked	1880
Salami	1800
Tomato ketchup	1630
Prawns, boiled	1590
Cheese, feta	1440
Butter	750
Houmous	670
Cheese, Cheddar	670
Digestive biscuits	660
Wholemeal bread	550
White bread	520
Sardines, canned in oil	450
Cottage cheese	380
Lobster, boiled	330
Scallops, steamed	180
Eggs, boiled	140
Yoghurt, low-fat, plain	83
Milk, skimmed and whole	55

Seafood is a natural source of sodium. Shellfish contain higher levels than fish, and fresh is best as a lot of canned seafood has sodium chloride added during processing.

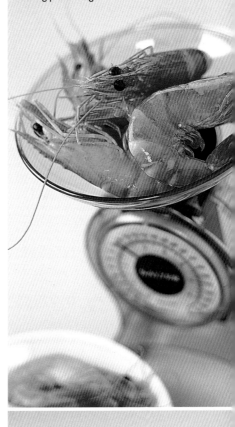

Most people, especially those suffering from high blood pressure, need to limit the amount of sodium in their diet. To achieve this, eliminate the use of table salt, buy salt-reduced products and keep a close eye on the amount of processed foods you eat.

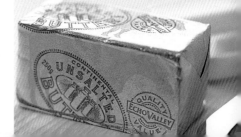

RECIPE Remove scallops from their shells and pan-fry in a little olive oil. Place some shredded fresh spinach on the cleaned shells, top with a scallop and serve with crumbled feta cheese and finely diced char-grilled marinated peppers.

Excessive perspiration, prolonged diarrhoea and vomiting increase the body's need for sodium. Electrolyte sports drinks are a simple way of gaining sodium. Contrary to popular belief, taking salt tablets will not stop cramps, so if you are healthy, don't take them. It is a lack of fluid that causes stitches and cramps.

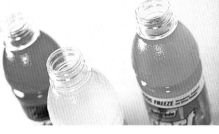

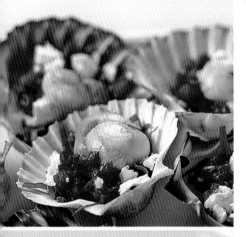

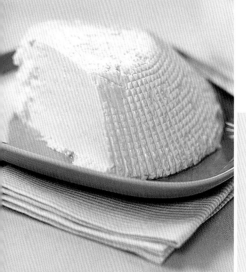

SODIUM works with potassium and chloride to regulate the acid and fluid balance in the body. It is necessary for proper muscle and nerve functioning and for maintaining a normal heartbeat. Table salt contains about 40 per cent sodium and 60 per cent chloride and its chemical name is sodium chloride. Most people in western countries eat more salt than they need and deficiency is rare.

Milk and dairy products contain relatively high levels of naturally occurring sodium so if you consume dairy products you really don't need to add salt to your meals.

CAUTION Currently in the UK we eat an average of 12 g salt every day. Our bodies need much less than this (about 4 g). Eating too much salt increases the amount of fluid that you retain in your body. This raises blood pressure – a major risk factor for heart disease and strokes. About three-quarters of our salt intake comes from processed foods, such as cured or smoked meats, meat products, bottled sauces and condiments, canned soups, processed cheese, crisps and salty snacks. Food labels do not usually give salt content, but the chemical name for salt is sodium chloride, and values for sodium are usually given on nutrition labels. 1 g of sodium is equivalent to about 1.5 g salt.

POTASSIUM

REFERENCE NUTRIENT INTAKE
Women and men: 3500 mg/day.

FOOD SOURCES	mg per 100 g
Yeast extract	2100
Dried yeast	2000
Apricots, dried	1880
Treacle, black	1760
Wheat bran	1160
Peaches, dried	1100
Sultanas	1060
Raisins	1020
Wheat germ	950
Pine nuts	780
Almonds	780
Parsley	760
Hazelnuts	730
Sunflower seeds	710
Dates, dried	700
Peanuts	760
Brazil nuts	660
Potatoes, baked with skin	630
Garlic	620
Coriander	540
Red snapper, fried	460
Avocados	450
Walnuts	450
Trout, rainbow, grilled	410
Bananas	400
Tempeh	370
Tuna, canned in oil	260
Yoghurt, plain	250
Carrots	170
Oranges	150
Milk, whole	140
Spinach, boiled	120
Apples	120

A cup of dried fruits is a simple way of getting your daily supply of potassium. Eaten as they are, or lightly simmered in apple juice, with spices, they make a tasty low-fat dessert or breakfast treat.

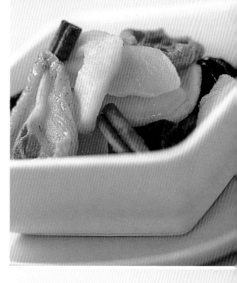

RECIPE Vegetarians can obtain generous amounts of potassium by including tempeh in their diets. It can be marinated in low-salt soy, garlic, ginger and then steamed, fried or barbecued and served on steamed greens.

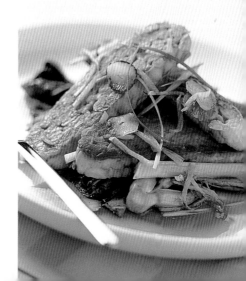

If you are prone to high blood pressure, decrease your sodium intake while increasing your potassium intake by eating more fruits and vegetables. Aim for at least five portions of fruit and vegetables every day.

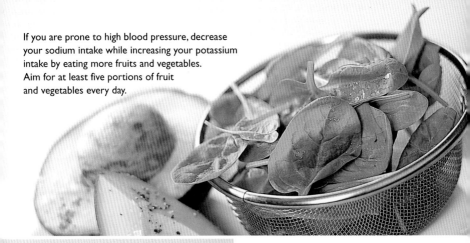

Bananas contain plenty of potassium so make them a part of your daily diet.

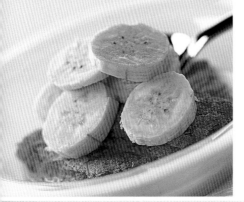

POTASSIUM, just like sodium, is necessary for maintaining the body's fluid balance, proper muscle and nerve function, and the metabolism of protein and carbohydrates. Potassium is present in many foods, so deficiency is unlikely. Potassium salt should not be used instead of table salt as a way of reducing sodium intake as it is very dangerous, especially for children.

RECIPE Seafood, especially snapper, is a rich source of potassium. Bake a whole snapper, then top it with a rich sauce of chopped herbs, pine nuts and garlic mixed with butter that has been combined with shredded lemon rind.

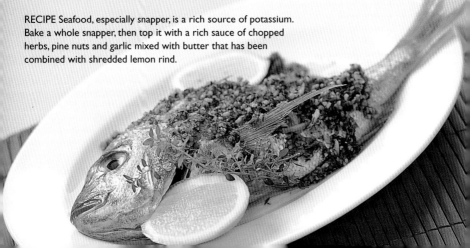

MINERALS – MAJOR
CHLORIDE

REFERENCE NUTRIENT INTAKE
Women and men: 2500 mg/day.

FOOD SOURCES	mg per 100 g
Salt	59900
Stock cubes	16000
Soy sauce	10640
Yeast extract	6630
Olives in brine	3750
Bacon back, grilled	2780
Prawns, boiled	2550
Cheese, Danish blue	1950
Cheese, Parmesan	1820
Cheese, Edam	1570
Cheese, Camembert	1120
Cheese, Cheddar	1030
Bread, white	820
Oysters	820
Sardines, canned in brine	810
Salmon, canned in brine	730
Peanuts, roasted and salted	660
Peanut butter	540
Tuna, canned in oil	530

Chlorine is often added to water for purification purposes as it prevents the growth of waterborne diseases, such as typhoid and hepatitis. Boiling the water evaporates the chlorine and may improve the taste.

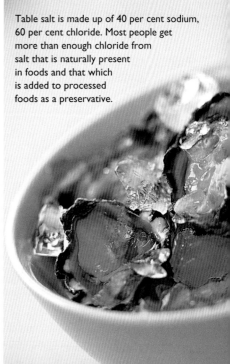

Table salt is made up of 40 per cent sodium, 60 per cent chloride. Most people get more than enough chloride from salt that is naturally present in foods and that which is added to processed foods as a preservative.

RECIPE Fill white bread with sliced Edam cheese, grilled bacon and a fried egg. Top with tomato sauce.

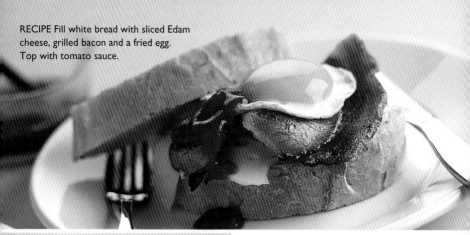

Chloride is combined with hydrogen in the stomach to make hydrochloric acid, which is essential for food digestion. Cheddar cheese is a good way to add chloride to your diet.

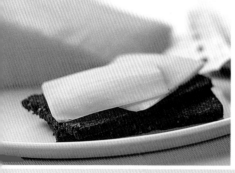

CHLORIDE, along with sodium and potassium, is important for maintaining the body's fluid balance and is therefore needed for normal muscle and nerve functioning. Virtually all of the chlorine found in foods and in our body is in the form of chloride. Deficiency is rare and only occurs when there are large losses through prolonged periods of vomiting, diarrhoea and profuse sweating.

Ripe olives stored in brine are a good way of getting chloride into your diet. Enjoy them on their own or add them to salads.

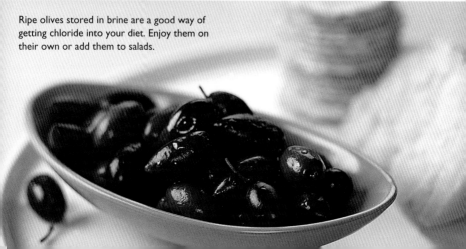

MINERALS – MAJOR
SULPHUR

No RNI. Most comes from the proteins we eat.

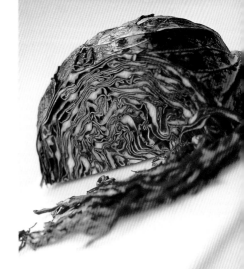

FOOD SOURCES	mcg per 100 g
Mustard powder	1280
Partridge, roast	400
Peanuts, plain	380
Cod, dried, salted, boiled	370
Peanut butter	360
Goose, roast	320
Bacon, gammon, lean, fried	310
Pork, loin, lean, grilled	310
Liver, calf, fried	300
Turkey, roast	290
Brazil nuts	290
Kidney, lamb, fried	290
Bacon, lean, grilled	290
Kipper, baked	280
Beef steak, lean, grilled	280
Mixed nuts	280
Liver, lamb, fried	270
Duck, roast	270
Chicken, lean, roast	260
Liver, chicken, fried	250
Cheese, Parmesan	250
Peaches, dried	240
Cheese, hard	230
Cheese, Stilton	230
Eggs, fried	200
Salmon, steamed	190
Egg, poached or boiled	180
Almonds	150
Walnuts	140
White bread rolls	130
Brussels sprouts	78
Red kidney beans	65
Red cabbage, boiled	54

Vegetarians who do not eat any eggs or dairy products can boost sulphur levels by eating nuts, beans and vegetables from the Brassica family, such as cabbage and Brussels sprouts.

RECIPE Cut pockets in chicken breast fillets, beat until thin with a mallet, then fill the pockets with Stilton cheese and pan-fry over medium heat until cooked through. Serve with steamed greens.

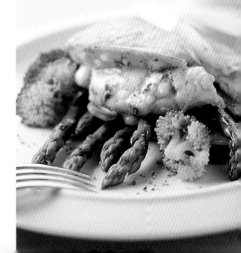

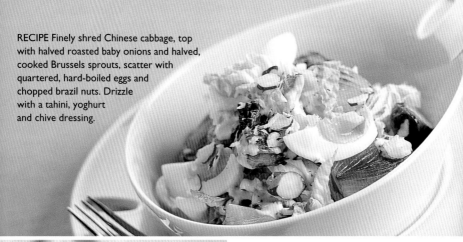

RECIPE Finely shred Chinese cabbage, top with halved roasted baby onions and halved, cooked Brussels sprouts, scatter with quartered, hard-boiled eggs and chopped brazil nuts. Drizzle with a tahini, yoghurt and chive dressing.

SULPHUR is known as the 'beauty mineral' as it is essential for healthy glossy skin, hair and nails. Sulphur helps regulate the acid/alkali balance in the body. Sulphur-containing amino acids are needed for protein synthesis, cell protection and detoxification.

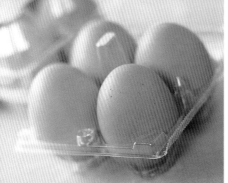

Protein-rich foods, especially eggs, meat and fish, are high in sulphur. If you have a diet with adequate protein you'll be meeting your sulphur requirements.

Sulphur-based creams and ointments may benefit those who suffer from skin problems such as psoriasis, eczema and dermatitis.

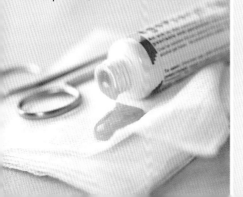

DEFICIENCY This is rare because we obtain most of our sulphur from proteins in the diet and it is also found in some preservatives.

CAUTION People who suffer from allergic reactions to food containing sulphur should avoid packaged dried fruit, which contains sulphur as a preservative. Look for sulphur-free varieties in health food stores.

MINERALS – TRACE
IRON

REFERENCE NUTRIENT INTAKE
Women 18 to 50 years: 14.8mg/day.
Women 50+ years: 8.7mg/day.
Men: 8.7mg/day.

FOOD SOURCES	mg per 100 g
Cockles, boiled	28
Black treacle	21.3
Fortified breakfast cereals	2–20
Seaweed, nori, dried	19.6
Wheat bran	19.2
Mussels, canned or bottled	13.0
Liver, calf, fried	12.2
Liver, chicken, fried	11.3
Kidney, lamb, fried	11.2
Liver, lamb, fried	10.9
Tahini	10.6
Cocoa powder	10.5
Sesame seeds	10.4
Winkles, boiled	10.2
Pumpkin seeds	10.4
Wheat germ	8.5
Meat extract	8.1
Clams, canned in brine	8.0
Parsley	7.7
Pâté, liver	7.4
Mussels, boiled	6.8
Peaches, dried	6.8
Sunflower seeds	6.4
Cashew nuts	6.2
Egg yolk	6.1
Lime pickle	5.8
Oysters	5.7
Pine nuts	5.6
Blackcurrants, canned in juice	5.2
Cous cous	5.0
Bulgar wheat	4.9

(continued)

Cooking for prolonged periods at high temperatures reduces the amount of iron in food, so choose cuts of meat or fish that can be steamed, poached or char-grilled, and try to get used to eating meat medium-rare.

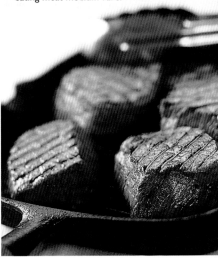

RECIPE Tofu provides some iron for vegetarians and can be enjoyed in a sweet or savoury meal. Serve silken firm tofu drizzled with a combination of sweet chilli sauce, sesame oil and soy sauce. Top with shredded, roasted nori.

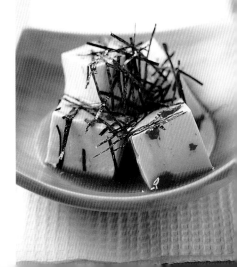

Because menstruating women can lose up to double the amount of iron in a month that men lose, it is essential they maintain adequate levels of iron in their diet. Mussels, clams, oysters and meat are all good sources of iron.

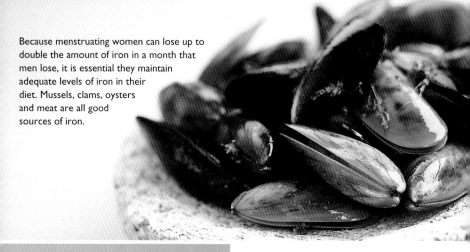

People who consume large quantities of tea or coffee need to be aware that they retard iron absorption. Substitute these with a fruit juice; it is high in vitamin C which increases absorption of iron.

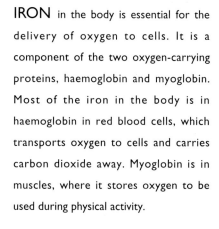

IRON in the body is essential for the delivery of oxygen to cells. It is a component of the two oxygen-carrying proteins, haemoglobin and myoglobin. Most of the iron in the body is in haemoglobin in red blood cells, which transports oxygen to cells and carries carbon dioxide away. Myoglobin is in muscles, where it stores oxygen to be used during physical activity.

Offal and red meat contain a form of iron (haem iron) that is easily absorbed by the body. Current healthy eating guidelines recommend that we eat a maximum of 90 g/day of red meat and processed meats.

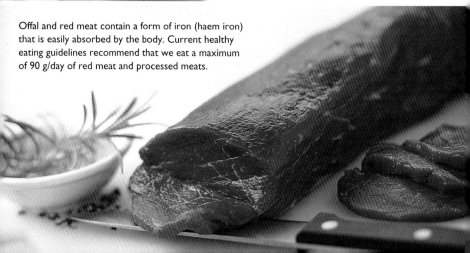

MINERALS – TRACE
IRON

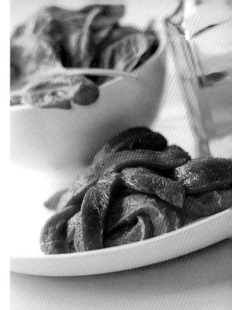

FOOD SOURCES (continued)	mg per 100 g
Miso	4.2
Apricots, dried	4.1
Raisins	3.8
Lentils, boiled	3.5
Tofu, steamed, fried	3.5
Hazelnuts	3.2
Sardines, canned in oil	3.1
Almonds	3.0
Soya beans, boiled	3.0
Walnuts	2.9
Prunes	2.9
Sardines, canned in tomato sauce	2.9
Wholemeal bread	2.7
Haricot beans, boiled	2.5
Peanut butter	2.5
Peanuts	2.5
Chocolate, plain	2.3
Swiss chard, boiled	2.3
Beef fillet, lean, grilled	2.3
Watercress	2.2
Eggs, fried	2.2
Sultanas	2.2
Spinach	2.1
Chickpeas, boiled	2.1
Curly kale, boiled	2.0
Red kidney beans, canned	2.0
Houmous	1.9
Eggs, boiled	1.9
Spinach, boiled	1.6
Peas, boiled	1.5
Pork fillet, lean, grilled	1.3
Broccoli, boiled	1.0
Tuna, canned in brine	1.0
Chicken, roast	0.7
Asparagus, boiled	0.6
Salmon, grilled	0.5
Brown rice, boiled	0.5

There are two types of iron in foods. Haem iron is in meat and meat products. Non-haem iron is in plant foods. Haem iron is much more readily absorbed than non-haem iron.

Foods containing vitamin C will increase iron absorption of non-haem iron so it is wise to include these foods with iron-rich meals. Try adding peppers to stir-fries and stews.

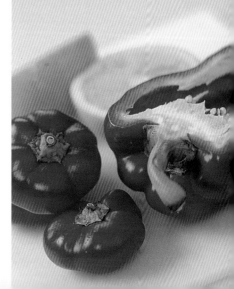

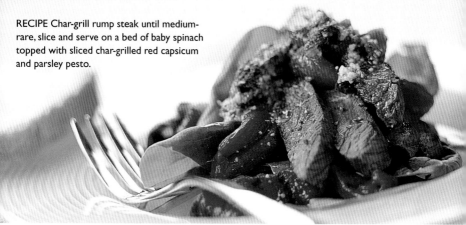

RECIPE Char-grill rump steak until medium-rare, slice and serve on a bed of baby spinach topped with sliced char-grilled red capsicum and parsley pesto.

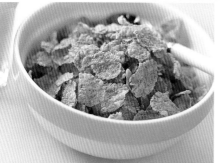

A bowl of muesli or iron-fortified breakfast cereal and a glass of orange juice each morning is a good start as the presence of vitamin C in the meal can enhance the absorption of iron.

IRON deficiency is the most common nutrient deficiency and many people have reduced iron stores. Deficiency impairs mood, ability to concentrate and physical performance, and can lead to anaemia. People who are most at risk of developing iron deficiency are women (particularly when pregnant), infants, fussy eaters, athletes and vegetarians.

Factors inhibiting iron absorption include phytates, calcium, soya protein and cooking at high temperature for prolonged periods. This doesn't mean you should avoid foods such as milk but try to have them separately from foods rich in iron.

DEFICIENCY Symptoms include fatigue, poor circulation, depression, reduced recovery from exercise, reduced physical and mental performance and anaemia.

CAUTION Never take high-dose supplements unless under medical supervision. People with haemochromatosis, which makes them absorb iron very efficiently, should not increase intake.

CAUTION Children under six years can mistake red iron supplements for sweets. Accidental overdose of just five pills leads to death, so store supplements away from children.

MINERALS – TRACE
ZINC

REFERENCE NUTRIENT INTAKE
Women: 7 mg/day.
(Lactation: 9.5 to 13 mg/day.)
Men: 9.5 mg/day.

FOOD SOURCES	mg per 100 g
Oysters	59.2
Wheat germ	17.0
Wheat bran	16.2
Liver, calf, fried	15.9
Whelks, boiled	12.1
Beef braising steak, lean, braised	9.5
Yeast, dried	8.0
Quorn myco-protein	7.5
Pumpkin seeds	6.6
Pine nuts	6.5
Liver, lamb, fried	5.9
Cashew nuts	5.9
Crab, canned in brine	5.7
Beef mince, extra lean, stewed	5.8
Crab, boiled	5.5
Pecan nuts	5.3
Cheese, Parmesan	5.3
Sesame seeds	5.3
Cheese, Emmental	4.4
Brazil nuts	4.2
Curry powder	4.1
Oat and wheat bran	4.0
Egg yolk	3.9
Kidney, lamb, fried	3.6
Miso	3.3
Anchovies, canned in oil	3.5
Pork fillet, lean, grilled	2.7
Cheese, Cheddar	2.3
Chicken, breast, grilled, no skin	0.8
Tofu, steamed	0.7
Milk, whole	0.4

RECIPE Children need zinc for normal growth. Adolescents who have acne may benefit from increasing the zinc in their diet. Prepare a burger with a wholewheat roll, lettuce, home-made minced steak, Cheddar cheese and tomato slices, grated carrot and fried egg.

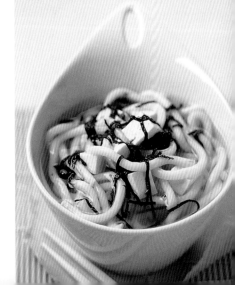

Vegetarians may struggle to find foods rich in zinc that is easily absorbed. A delicious miso udon noodle soup topped with shredded nori and cubed tofu will help with zinc intake.

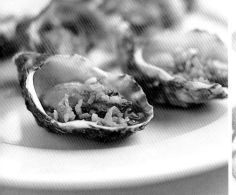

Oysters win hands down when it comes to zinc. Enjoy them natural or topped with your favourite sauce and grilled.

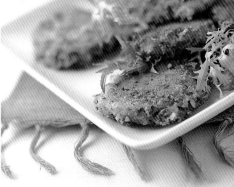

RECIPE Prepare crab cakes using canned crab, mashed potato, a pinch of curry powder, fresh herbs and grated Cheddar cheese.

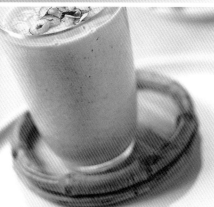

RECIPE In your blender, make a drink using skimmed milk powder, oat bran, wheat germ, hazelnuts and fresh mango.

ZINC wears many hats. It is required to assist our appetite as well as our sense of smell and taste. It helps fight infections, improves immunity, maintains healthy nails, skin, hair, tissue growth and repair, and is necessary for sexual development and reproduction. Zinc is involved in the action of many enzymes that control various chemical reactions in the body.

Beef is one of the best dietary sources of zinc. Spaghetti bolognese or a beef stir-fry are delicious ways to keep it in the diet.

DEFICIENCY Signs are loss of taste, smell and appetite, poor growth and wound healing, reduced libido and sperm count, late onset of puberty, dry flaky skin, dandruff, and increased susceptibility to infection. People at risk of deficiency include alcoholics, vegans, children and elderly people with poor diets.

CAUTION Zinc supplements can result in toxicity problems such as gastrointestinal irritation, decreased immunity and reduced copper absorption. Supplements containing more than 50 mg of elemental zinc should be avoided as they may cause nausea, headaches and decreased copper absorption.

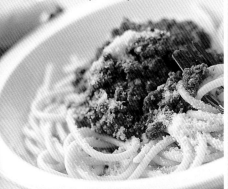

MINERALS – TRACE
COPPER

REFERENCE NUTRIENT INTAKE
Women and men: 1.2mg/day.
(Lactation: 1.5mg/day.)

FOOD SOURCES	mg per 100 g
Liver, calf, fried	23.9
Liver, lamb, fried	13.5
Oysters	7.5
Whelks, boiled	6.6
Dried yeast	5.0
Cocoa powder	3.9
Tomato puree	2.9
Sunflower seeds	2.3
Cashew nuts	2.1
Shrimps, boiled	1.9
Crab, boiled	1.8
Brazil nuts	1.8
Winkles, boiled	1.7
Pumpkin seeds	1.6
Sesame seeds	1.5
Tahini	1.5
Lobster, boiled	1.4
Walnuts	1.3
Pine nuts	1.3
Hazelnuts	1.2
Pecan nuts	1.1
Peanuts	1.0
Squid	1.0
Almonds	1.0
Curry powder	1.0
Pistachio nuts, roasted, salted	0.8
Quorn myco-protein	0.8
Currants	0.8
Peanut butter	0.7
Tempeh	0.7
Mushrooms	0.7
Peaches, dried	0.6

RECIPE Fill a sesame seed wholemeal roll with tempeh. Marinate tempeh pieces with a little dressing made by mixing balsamic vinegar, sunflower oil, crushed garlic and tahini. Season with cracked black pepper. Char-grill and serve with salad greens.

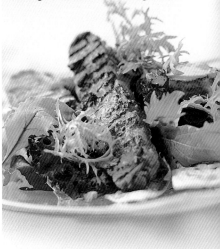

RECIPE Simmer tempeh in a lightly spiced coconut curry with cashew nuts and your choice of vegetables.

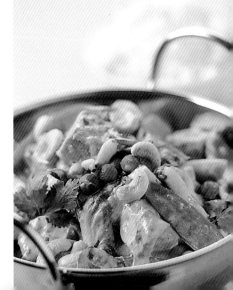

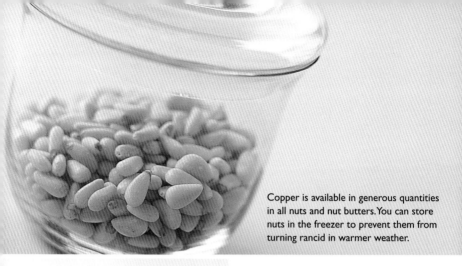

Copper is available in generous quantities in all nuts and nut butters. You can store nuts in the freezer to prevent them from turning rancid in warmer weather.

Oysters are a source of copper, although the levels can vary depending on where they are grown. Cooked oysters have nearly twice as much copper as the raw ones.

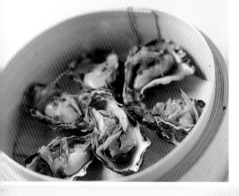

COPPER assists the body in the metabolism of iron and fat. It is required to maintain the heart muscle and tissue and the immune and central nervous systems. Copper is also involved in the formation of melanin and is important for healthy hair and skin. Deficiency is rare, but causes decreased immunity, anaemia, osteoporosis and degeneration of the heart muscle and nervous system.

RECIPE Stir-fry cleaned, honeycombed squid pieces with plenty of crushed garlic, shredded ginger and peanut oil until the squid turns white. Add sliced spring onion and a few generous splashes of sweet chilli sauce and fresh lime.

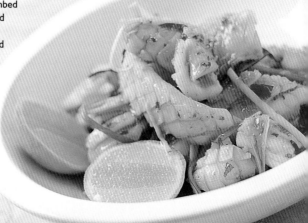

MINERALS – TRACE
MANGANESE

SAFE INTAKE
Adults: more than 1.4 mg/day.

FOOD SOURCES	mg per 100 g
Wheat germ	12.3
Wheat bran	9.0
Pine nuts	7.9
Seaweed, nori, dried	6.0
Macadamia nuts, salted	5.5
Hazelnuts	4.9
Pecan nuts	4.6
Oatmeal	3.7
Mushrooms, oyster	3.6
Crispbread, rye	3.5
Pineapple, dried	3.4
Walnuts	3.4
Muesli, no added sugar	2.6
Sunflower seeds	2.2
Quorn myco-protein	2.1
Peanuts	2.1
Wholemeal bread	1.9
Peanut butter	1.8
Almonds	1.7
Cashew nuts	1.7
Sesame seeds	1.5
Blackberries	1.4
Coconut cream	1.3
Pasta, wholemeal, boiled	0.9
Rice, brown, boiled	0.9
Pineapple, canned in juice	0.9
Watercress	0.6
White bread	0.5
Sweet potato, baked	0.5
Spinach, boiled	0.5
Houmous	0.5
Apples, dried	0.5
Red kidney beans, boiled	0.5
Mussels, canned or bottled	0.5

RECIPE Steam mussels in some white wine with chopped fresh lemon grass and chopped tomato. Mop up the delicious juice with wholemeal bread.

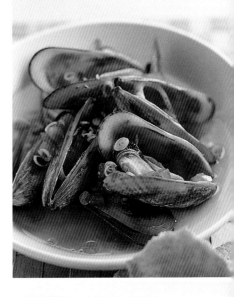

RECIPE For a delicious milkshake, process blackberries, wheat germ, hazelnuts, coconut cream and milk in a blender.

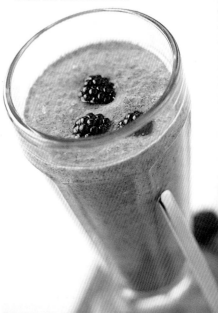

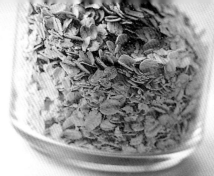

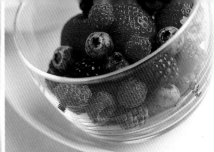

Although manganese occurs naturally in whole grains and cereals, up to 90 per cent can be removed in the milling process, so choose whole grains that have not been subjected to unnecessary amounts of processing.

Add manganese to your diet by snacking on fresh berries in season. Mixed with ice and a little fruit juice, they make a refreshing summer drink.

Good dietary sources are nuts, seeds and wholegrain cereals. Make up a nut and seed praline that can be eaten as a snack or crumbled and served over ice cream.

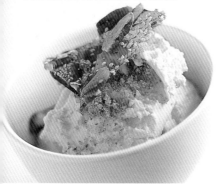

MANGANESE has quite a varied role in the body. It has been found to be an effective antioxidant. It is necessary for the formation of bone and sex hormones and is also involved in carbohydrate and fat metabolism, as well as proper brain functioning. Deficiency is rare and unlikely in normal circumstances.

Large quantities of manganese can be found in all types of seaweed. To add manganese to the diet, try sprinkling shredded roasted seaweed (nori) on rice or salads.

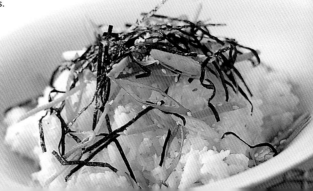

MINERALS – TRACE
IODINE

REFERENCE NUTRIENT INTAKE
Women and men: 140 mcg/day.
Exact figures for iodine in foods are difficult to
establish but good food sources are listed below.

FOOD SOURCES

Bread
Butter
Peppers (capsicum), green
Cereals
Cheese, Cheddar
Clams
Cod
Cottage cheese
Crab
Cream
Dairy products
Eggs
Fruits
Haddock
Lettuce
Lobster
Meat
Milk
Mussels
Oysters
Peanuts
Pineapple
Prawns
Raisins
Salmon
Salt, iodised
Sardines
Seaweed
Spinach
Tuna, canned
Vegetables

Seafood and deep-water fish such as cod,
halibut, salmon and haddock are excellent
sources of this mineral. Plant foods grown
in soil by the sea absorb iodine from the
sea spray.

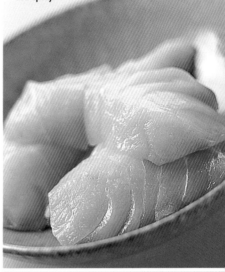

RECIPE Coat salmon fillets in sesame seeds,
wrap with a wide strip of roasted nori and
brush the edges lightly to seal. Pan-fry
until tender and serve with steamed rice
and mayonnaise.

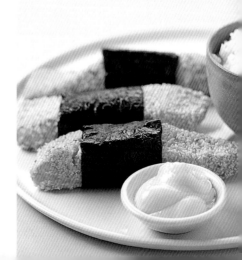

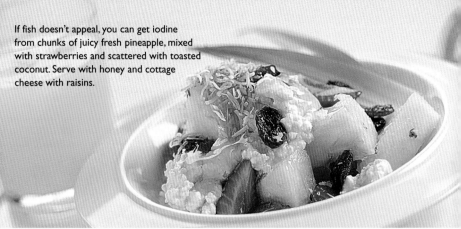

If fish doesn't appeal, you can get iodine from chunks of juicy fresh pineapple, mixed with strawberries and scattered with toasted coconut. Serve with honey and cottage cheese with raisins.

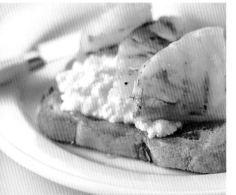

IODINE is essential for the production of the hormones produced by the thyroid gland, which regulate the body's metabolic rate, growth and development, and promote protein synthesis. Selenium is also needed for the synthesis of the thyroid hormones.

RECIPE Fruit bread topped with sweetened cottage cheese and fried slices of pineapple.

Because iodine levels in the soil in some regions are low, iodine is added to salt and is sold as iodised salt. If you have a low-salt diet you may need to monitor your iodine requirements. Deficiency is rare in Western societies because of the relatively high intake of salt.

DEFICIENCY Rare in Western societies, deficiency reduces thyroid hormone production and leads to a lowered metabolic rate, which leads to tiredness and weight gain and the thyroid gland becoming enlarged (goitre). If iodine is deficient in pregnancy, there is a greater risk of stillbirth and miscarriage and of mental retardation and growth failure in the baby.

CAUTION Excessive intake of iodine (30 times the RNI) may result in mouth sores, swollen salivary glands, diarrhoea, vomiting, headaches and difficulty breathing. It can lead to goitre, although goitre is more common if the body is iodine deficient.

MINERALS – TRACE
CHROMIUM

SAFE INTAKE
Adults: more than 25 mcg/day.

FOOD SOURCES	mcg per 100 g*
Egg yolk	183
Brewer's yeast	112
Beef	57
Cheese, Cheddar	56
Liver, all types	55
Wine, white/red	45
Bread, wholegrain	42
Black pepper	35
Bread, rye	30
Chilli	30
Apple peel	27
Potatoes, old	27
Oysters	26
Potatoes, new	21
Margarine	18
Spaghetti	15
Spirits	14
Butter	13
Spinach	10
Egg white	8
Oranges	5
Beer	3–30
Apple, peeled	1

Elderly people with diets high in refined foods may be in danger of becoming deficient in chromium because chromium is lost during the milling of grains. Eat wholegrain instead of white bread and use wholemeal flour instead of white.

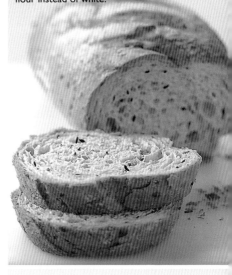

RECIPE Toss cooked spaghetti with shredded fresh spinach, chopped chilli, cracked pepper, toasted wholemeal breadcrumbs and butter.

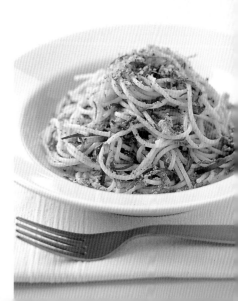

*Australian values.

RECIPE Serve thick slices of wholegrain bread topped with baby spinach leaves, barbecued thin beef steaks and barbecued onions and mushrooms. Top with a dollop of sour cream flavoured with honey mustard. Serve with potato wedges.

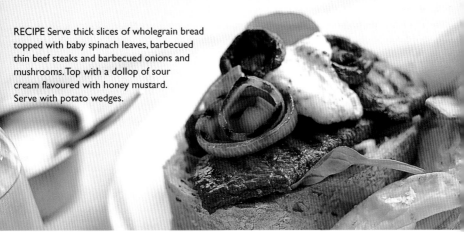

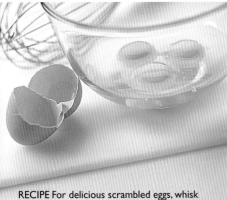

RECIPE For delicious scrambled eggs, whisk some eggs, add plenty of grated Cheddar and cook the mixture in melted butter. Spinach is an ideal accompaniment.

CHROMIUM is essential for the hormone, insulin, to function properly, and is therefore involved in maintaining blood sugar levels. Deficiency is uncommon, but can occur in undernourished elderly people and children with very poor diets. Symptoms include high blood glucose and insulin levels and possibly high blood cholesterol and triglyceride levels.

If you cook with stainless steel cookware, the chromium from the steel is leached into the food and therefore your chromium intake is increased.

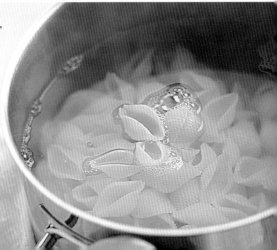

MINERALS – TRACE
MOLYBDENUM

SAFE INTAKE
Adults: 50–400 mcg/day.
Exact figures for molybdenum are difficult to
establish, listed below are good food sources.

FOOD SOURCES

Apricots

Barley

Beef

Bread, rye

Bread, wholemeal

Cabbage

Carrots

Cauliflower

Cereal grains

Cheese

Chicken

Coconut

Corn

Crab

Eggs

Garlic

Kidneys

Lamb

Legumes

Lentils

Liver, all types

Melon, cantaloupe-type

Milk

Oats, rolled

Onion

Peas, green

Potatoes

Raisins

Rice, brown

Spinach

Sunflower seeds

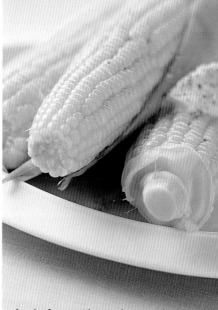

A cob of corn with some butter melted
over the top served with your evening
meal is a simple and tasty way to add
some molybdenum to your diet.

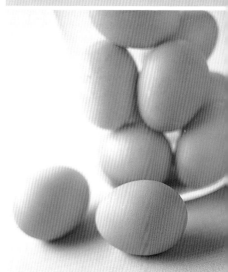

The quantity of molybdenum is largely
dependent on the amount occurring in the
soil that foods are grown in. Processing can
also reduce molybdenum in foods. Eggs are
less susceptible to soil variation and the diets
of chickens are regularly monitored.

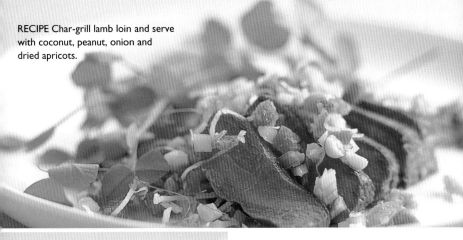

RECIPE Char-grill lamb loin and serve with coconut, peanut, onion and dried apricots.

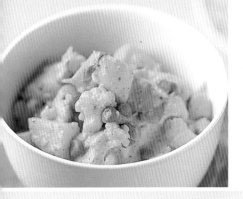

A potato, pea and cauliflower curry in coconut milk, served with brown rice is a good way of adding molybdenum to the diet.

MOLYBDENUM is necessary to activate certain major enzymes in the body. These enzymes are needed for DNA synthesis and for the production of uric acid. Molybdenum is also important for the production of waste products so they can be excreted from the body. Deficiency is rare and unlikely to occur under normal conditions.

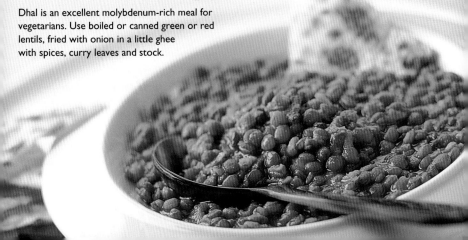

Dhal is an excellent molybdenum-rich meal for vegetarians. Use boiled or canned green or red lentils, fried with onion in a little ghee with spices, curry leaves and stock.

MINERALS – TRACE
FLUORIDE

No RNI or safe intake for adults.
Fluoride figures are difficult to establish but foods containing fluoride are listed below.

FOOD SOURCES

Apples
Asparagus
Barley
Beetroot
Cabbage
Cheese, Cheddar
Corn
Fish, fresh
Fish, canned
Fruits, citrus
Garlic
Kale
Milk, goat's
Milk, skimmed
Millet
Oats
Rice
Rice bran
Salt, sea
Seafood
Spinach
Tea
Water, fluoridated
Watercress

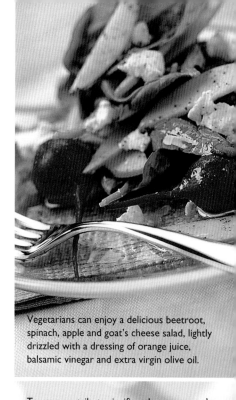

Vegetarians can enjoy a delicious beetroot, spinach, apple and goat's cheese salad, lightly drizzled with a dressing of orange juice, balsamic vinegar and extra virgin olive oil.

Tea can contribute significantly to a person's fluoride intake if they drink a lot, depending on the amount of dry leaves used, brewing time and the fluoride content in the water.

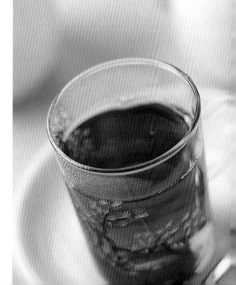

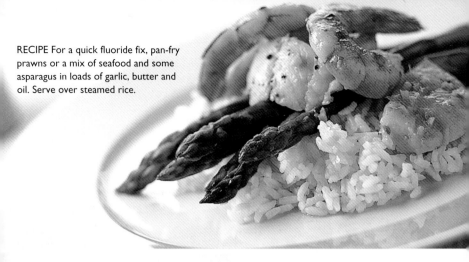

RECIPE For a quick fluoride fix, pan-fry prawns or a mix of seafood and some asparagus in loads of garlic, butter and oil. Serve over steamed rice.

People who choose not to drink water containing fluoride can obtain the mineral by incorporating seafood in their diet.

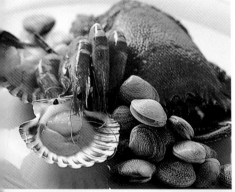

FLUORIDE is contained in every bone in our bodies as well as teeth. It reduces our chances of tooth decay and discolouration. This is why it is added to toothpaste and drinking water. Fluoride may also keep our bones strong. Some people believe that fluoridated water causes health problems, but these claims are not supported by any evidence.

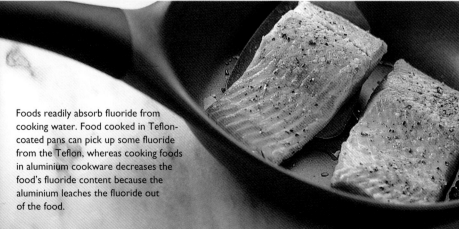

Foods readily absorb fluoride from cooking water. Food cooked in Teflon-coated pans can pick up some fluoride from the Teflon, whereas cooking foods in aluminium cookware decreases the food's fluoride content because the aluminium leaches the fluoride out of the food.

MINERALS – TRACE
SELENIUM

REFERENCE NUTRIENT INTAKE
Women: 60 mcg/day. (Lactation: 75 mcg/day.)
Men: 75mcg/day.

FOOD SOURCES	mcg per 100 g
Brazil nuts	1530
Kidney, pig, fried	270
Mixed nuts and raisins	170
Lobster, boiled	130
Tuna, canned in oil	90
Kidney, lamb, fried	88
Lemon sole, steamed	73
Squid	66
Mullet, red, grilled	54
Scallops, steamed	51
Sardines, canned in oil	49
Sunflower seeds	49
Herring, grilled	46
Shrimps, boiled	46
Plaice, grilled	45
Mussels, boiled	43
Kipper, baked	43
Mackerel, canned in brine	42
Wholemeal bread	35
Cod, baked	34
Salmon, grilled	31
Scone, wholemeal, fruit	31
Crumpets	24
Prawns, boiled	23
Houmous	23
Oysters	23
Pork fillet, lean, grilled	21
Egg yolk	20
Crab, boiled	17
Chicken breast, grilled, no skin	16
Cheese, Cheddar,	12
Eggs, fried	12

Brazil nuts are right at the top of the list as a source of selenium. Eat them as a snack or chop some and serve over your favourite ice cream.

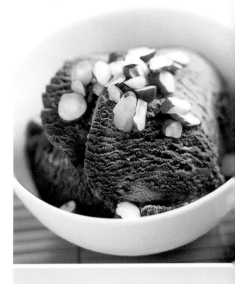

RECIPE Wholemeal bread sandwiches for children, spread with hummus and topped with canned tuna and salad greens, will ensure their selenium requirements are met.

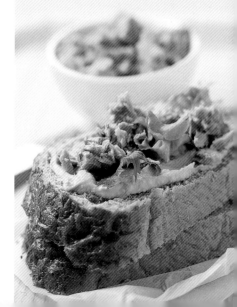

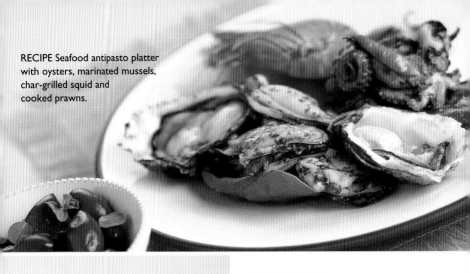

RECIPE Seafood antipasto platter with oysters, marinated mussels, char-grilled squid and cooked prawns.

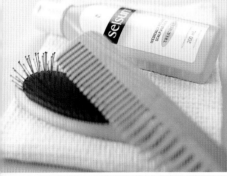

Selenium is easily absorbed through the skin and selenium-based shampoos are extremely effective in the treatment of dandruff or dry scalp.

SELENIUM is best known for its antioxidant properties and works with vitamin E to protect the body against free radicals. Selenium is also essential for the production of thyroid hormones that regulate the metabolic rate in our bodies and may help protect us from heart disease. Selenium deficiency is rare. Do not take daily supplements that contain more than 200 mcg. Toxic symptoms include nervousness, depression, nausea, vomiting and loss of hair and fingernails.

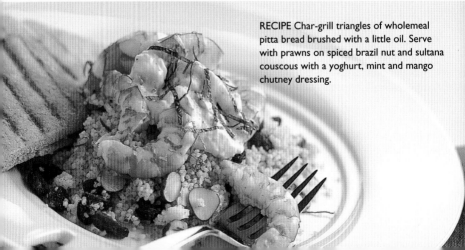

RECIPE Char-grill triangles of wholemeal pitta bread brushed with a little oil. Serve with prawns on spiced brazil nut and sultana couscous with a yoghurt, mint and mango chutney dressing.

BIBLIOGRAPHY

Kirschmann, John & Gayla, *Nutrition Almanac*, 4th edition, McGraw Hill, 1996.

Mindell, Earl, *The Vitamin Bible*, Arlington Books, 1982.

Osiecki, Henry, *Nutrients in Profile,* Bioconcepts Publishing, 1990.

Saxelby, Catherine, *Nutrition for Life*, Reed, 1993.

Scott-Moncrieff, Christina Dr, *The Vitamin Alphabet*, Simon & Schuster, 1999.

Shils, Maurice E. and Young, Vernon, R. (editors), *Modern Nutrition in Health and Disease*, 7th edition, Lea & Bebiger, 1988.

Smolin, Lori A. and Grosvenor, Mary B., *Nutrition Science and Applications*, 3rd edition, Saunders Collegé Publishing, 2000.

Stanton, Rosemary, *Eating for Peak Performance*, 2nd editon, Allen & Unwin, 1994.

Urs, Koch Manfred, *Laugh with Health*, Renaissance and New Age Creations, 1981.

Current UK guidelines for intakes of nutrients are drawn from the Committee on Medical Aspects of Food Policy's (COMA) Panel on Dietary Reference Values, which published its report *Dietary Reference Values for Food and Energy and Nutrients in the UK* in 1991.